The Sleep Workbook

The
SLEEP
WORKBOOK

EASY STRATEGIES to BREAK
the ANXIETY-INSOMNIA CYCLE

RENATA ALEXANDRE, PHD

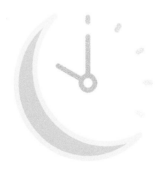

ROCKRIDGE
PRESS

Interior & Cover Designer: Brian Lewis
Art Producer: Hannah Dickerson
Editor: Meera Pal
Production Editor: Matt Burnett

Art courtesy of Shutterstock and Creative Market. Icons made by Freepik from flaticon.com
Author photograph courtesy of Ascension Health

ISBN: Print 978-1-64611-631-7 | eBook 978-1-64611-632-4

Ro

This book is dedicated to all of the patients who have entrusted their insomnia care to me, as well as to my colleagues and my staff from whom I learn something new every day. Most of all, I would like to dedicate this book to Kelly Carden, MD, who taught me most of what I know about sleep medicine and has been my guide on this journey.

CONTENTS

· · · ·

INTRODUCTION

For most of my life, I have been a poor sleeper. I couldn't take naps in kinder-garten, and I was usually the last to go to sleep and one of the first to wake up during childhood sleepovers. My inability to sleep caused me to have major anxiety. My mind would race in the night while I lay awake in bed, and I became an expert catastrophizer. In my teens, I had difficulty going to bed before midnight and getting up before 10 a.m. In my twenties, I had difficulty being at work on time when I worked the day shift. My favorite shift as an RN was the evening shift (3 to 11 p.m.).

By my 30s and 40s, I had resigned myself to being a sleepy person. I developed some coping mechanisms and learned that if I awakened early, sometimes I could go back to bed an hour later and get more sleep. But, inev-itably, I felt more tired when I did that. When I went back to college in my 40s, the long hours of studying did not allow for sleep. I actually did better with sleep during that time because I was spending less time in bed, but I did not connect the dots.

After I earned my PhD, I was offered the opportunity to become a CBT-I specialist at a sleep center, and I began to learn about sleep. I was having difficulty with my sleep, so my mentor did a few sessions of CBT-I with me. To my surprise, we discovered that I am actually a 4.5-to-5-hour sleeper.

After two weeks of sessions, I was feeling better. After two months, I had improved even more, and I have been pretty stable since a year after our first session. I now spend 5.5 to 6 hours in bed, and I get to sleep quickly and stay asleep very easily. Of course, I am still a night owl, but I've developed a morning routine that gives me the vitality I need for the day. Life is good, and I have the energy to do what I want to do most of the time. Yes, I still have an anxious night now and then, but it's become a rare occurrence.

I tell this story because I would like you to experience the same success in treatment as I have. I won't deceive you and say it's easy because it's not. But every effort you put into the process will be rewarded as long as you remain patient and persistent. You can change your sleep and decrease your anxiety. And, in the process, you'll likely develop greater self-confidence because you were able to help yourself. Persistence is key to resolving sleep and anxiety issues. I wish you the best in your search for refreshing sleep and a calm mind.

PART ONE

· · · · · · · · · · · ·

SLEEP
101

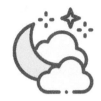

CHAPTER ONE

Sleep, Insomnia, Anxiety

· · ·

Suffering with both insomnia and anxiety is common because they are inter-related; anxiety can make it difficult to sleep, and lack of sleep can worsen anxiety symptoms. In this chapter, we will explore how the body responds to anxiety and insomnia and how cognitive behavioral therapy (CBT) can help you change the way you think, improve your life, and get a good night's sleep.

THE IMPORTANCE OF SLEEP ······················

More than one-third of adults in the United States typically obtain less than the recommended seven to nine hours of sleep per night. As a culture, we tend to value hard work over quality sleep. So, when the demands of our work, family, and personal lives exceed the time there is in a day to get it all done, we tend to sacrifice sleep. To many of us, it's the one thing that can be forfeited so that we can spend more time doing other tasks. A 2019 article on BBC.com noted that sleep is habitually taken for granted and under-valued. But as we learn more about the benefits of sleep, we're recognizing how important it is for our well-being. In fact, this understanding has led to laws that require certain public workers to have an adequate amount of qual-ity sleep before their shifts. For instance, truck drivers and pilots are now screened and required to undergo sleep studies if they show indications of sleep apnea.

When we are awake, the chemical processes in our body that allow us to function at our best become depleted. Sleep allows our bodies to restore these processes and function at an ideal level. During sleep, our bodies undergo sev-eral critical tasks, including memory consolidation (both cognitive and muscle memory), brain temperature regulation, energy conservation, restoration of neurochemicals, hormonal regulation, and other neurocognitive functions.

Research shows that sleep is critical to our physical and mental health. Over time, a lack of sleep can lead to a drop in physical performance, a weaker immune system, cognitive decline, cardiovascular disease, hyper-tension, obesity, and substance abuse, as well as a host of mood disorders. In addition, those suffering from inadequate sleep are less likely to recognize their impairments.

Studies also show that the cognitive and motor impairment seen in those suffering from sleep deprivation is equivalent to those with blood alcohol levels above the legal limit. A study by the AAA Foundation for Traffic Safety found that driving drowsy results in an estimated 328,000 traffic collisions a year. Sleepiness also has a significant impact on learning, memory, grades, and mood.

As you can see, sleep is vital for our bodies to function properly. Adequate sleep is not a luxury—it's a necessity. Sleep disorders can have a serious effect on your health.

Sleepiness vs. Fatigue

The words sleepiness and fatigue are often used interchangeably, but there's a significant difference between the two. Sleepiness refers to your ability to fall asleep easily, even during the day. If you are significantly sleepy and you are able to relax for a moment, you can nod off to sleep without difficulty. Fatigue refers to a lack of energy or motivation. Someone suffering from fatigue is rarely able to sleep outside their scheduled sleep time.

As a sleep clinician, one of the questions I ask to determine whether someone is sleepy or fatigued is if they find it easy to nap during the day. Most individuals with insomnia find it very difficult to nap because they are likely not sleepy but fatigued. If someone is able to nap easily during the day, my concern becomes ruling out another underlying sleep fragmentation disorder.

PRIMARY TYPES OF INSOMNIA

The American Academy of Sleep Medicine defines insomnia as "a persistent difficulty with sleep initiation, duration, consolidation, or quality that occurs despite adequate opportunity and circumstances for sleep and results in some form of daytime impairment." The three major components of insomnia include:

- Adequate opportunity to obtain sleep
- Difficulty with sleep
- Problems with daytime function as a result of poor sleep

Those with insomnia have difficulty getting to sleep and staying asleep. Sometimes, they will also wake up early in the morning and be unable to return to sleep. Someone experiencing insomnia typically complains of daytime sleepiness but is still unable to nap.

Short sleepers often believe they have insomnia, but that is not necessarily the case. There are those who need less sleep than the seven-to-nine-hour average, which is normal. Short sleepers can sleep fewer than seven to eight hours with no daytime effects. When short sleepers spend too much time in bed, they are often as tired as someone who doesn't spend enough time in bed. This is because their sleep becomes fragmented and, therefore, of lower quality.

There are several types of insomnia:

Acute Insomnia

Anything that causes stress can lead to acute insomnia. Acute insomnia is frequently associated with an event or stressor that has occurred in an individual's life. Often, these are life-changing events like the loss of a loved one, a move or change in location, or a change in employment. Shifts in personal relationships—such as divorce, a disagreement with a loved one, or changes in work relationships—can also cause insomnia. Acute insomnia is generally short-term and resolves with time, but people who have anxiety or depression may be more prone to acute insomnia.

Chronic Insomnia

Chronic insomnia refers to persistent delay of sleep, fragmented sleep, or both. The hallmark of chronic insomnia is "performance anxiety." In other words, when someone knows they regularly have difficulty with sleep. They begin to worry about their ability to get to sleep, stay asleep, or both. These individuals may also find it much easier to sleep away from home because their own bed has become a battleground of sorts.

Comorbid Insomnia

Comorbid refers to other behavioral or health problems that are frequently seen with insomnia. These can include attitudes and behaviors that prevent sleep, habitual practices that interfere with optimal sleep, as well as painful conditions that hinder sleep. It can also be related to medications like water pills (which can make you need to use the bathroom during the night), prednisone, or other stimulating medications that make sleep difficult.

Delayed Onset

We refer to people who like to stay awake late into the night and rise later in the day as night owls. These people often have a delay in melatonin production, so the stimulus that helps them get to sleep does not occur until later in the day. This is a natural phenomenon for some people.

Fragmented Sleep

This refers to difficulty staying asleep. Short sleepers frequently experience fragmented sleep because their sleep drive is short. If they spend too much time in bed, the drive for sleep is reduced, and they wake up frequently for significant periods of time in the night. Someone with comorbid insomnia may suffer from fragmented sleep. It's more difficult to wake up feeling refreshed when sleep is fragmented.

Insomnia Statistics

Insomnia affects about 30 percent of the United States population, according to a 2016 issue of Journal of Family Medicine and Primary Care. *Most often, conditions that are present with insomnia are psychiatric—anxiety, depression, and mood and personality disorders. Insomnia generally occurs more often in females than males.*

Delayed onset sleep is a condition most frequently seen in adolescence, but adults with a strong biological clock may experience symptoms well into their later years. Arminoff's Neurology and General Medicine, 5th Edition, *revealed that the prevalence in the population of adults with delayed onset sleep is 0.17 percent. In the insomnia subset of the population, the prevalence of delayed onset sleep is 5 to 10 percent.*

Sleep Disorders

Sleep disorders can contribute to insomnia through sleep fragmentation, difficulty getting to sleep, or sleep maintenance. Some of the most common sleep disorders are described below. If you have one of these disorders, you may want to discuss your symptoms with your primary care provider.

Obstructive Sleep Apnea (OSA)

Obstructive sleep apnea occurs when the tongue and soft tissue of the mouth relax into the back of the throat multiple times per hour, closing the airway. Oxygen levels in the bloodstream decrease, and the brain uses the stress hormones to wake the body in order to start breathing again. Consequently, sleep becomes fragmented, and daytime tiredness is common. Symptoms include snoring, witnessed apnea (stopped breathing), and waking up as a result of choking and gasping during sleep.

Restless Legs Syndrome (RLS)

Restless legs syndrome is a tremendous urge to move the legs, typically occurring in the evening. It is often accompanied by an uncomfortable sensation in the legs that is frequently described as a creepy, crawly feeling. Movement helps, but the symptoms usually return once you are still again. Symptoms typically begin when the body is at rest. RLS can also cause sleep fragmentation if it occurs in the night. Most frequently, this issue contributes to sleep-onset insomnia.

Circadian Sleep Wake Disorders (CSWD)

Circadian sleep wake disorders are characterized by a mismatch between the inborn biological sleep-wake rhythm (biological clock, also known as your circadian clock) and the timing of sleep, daytime activities, and social activities. Common CSWDs include shift-work disorder, jet lag, and delayed onset sleep. People with strong biological clocks have difficulty adapting to social and environmental cues that tell them it's time to sleep or wake up. This can result in difficulty getting to sleep, staying asleep, and waking at desired times.

SELF-REFLECTION

Have you experienced any of the symptoms discussed under "Sleep Disorders"? Write down what you have experienced. Do they align with any of the disorders on page 9?

_____

_____

_____

_____

_____

UNDERSTANDING ANXIETY

Anxiety is characterized by a feeling of apprehension or uneasiness and is usually brought on by a trigger that isn't a real threat. Anxiety can manifest in several ways, both physically and cognitively.

Anxiety and Your Body

Individuals may have inherited a tendency toward anxious behaviors. Anxiety can also be learned from family members as a way of coping with stressors. Our bodies respond to stress in various ways. Someone who is regularly exposed to stress can develop anxiety or fear as a learned response to repeated threats. The person's perception of a given situation is moderated by age, experience, gender, the environment, specific characteristics of the triggering event, and personality qualities. If you have anxiety, there was a point in your life when your ability to adapt to stress was compromised. You are left with feelings of fear and anxiety when triggers are activated.

It is important to discuss anxiety symptoms with your primary care provider if they are causing you to experience stress on a daily basis. Failing to do so can worsen other disease processes that also trigger the stress response, thereby worsening both the anxiety and other conditions.

The brain does not distinguish between a physical threat and a psychological threat, so the response is the same. The body secretes stress hormones—adrenaline and cortisol—into the bloodstream to cope with the stressor. During the stress response, the body shuts down the systems it does not need and activates those systems that will be required to either fight if there is a confrontation or flee to safety. Digestion slows, which may manifest as choking, dry mouth, and nausea. The heart rate increases, which elevates your blood pressure. Blood flow to your large muscles increases, and you may become hyper-alert and experience excessive sweating and a flushed face or body. You also breathe faster to get plenty of oxygen to the muscles to prepare for fleeing the situation.

Anxiety and Your Brain

The imbalance of four primary neurotransmitters (chemical messengers in the brain) is usually present in anxiety.

1. Dopamine is associated with pleasure, learning, and motivation. Too much dopamine can cause delusive thinking and punishing thoughts.

2. Serotonin affects your mood, appetite, and sleep. It is believed to regulate anxiety and reduce depression.

3. Gamma-aminobutyric acid (GABA) inhibits neuronal activity and is thought to produce a calming effect on the brain and nervous system.

4. Adrenaline excites the brain and body, increasing the heart rate, blood flow to the muscles, and alertness. It is secreted when the brain senses a threat.

When we are under stress, the imbalance of these neurotransmitters is thought to increase the likelihood of experiencing anxiety symptoms. Patients with anxiety typically have lower levels of serotonin and GABA; a shortage of these neurotransmitters causes higher levels of dopamine activity. In the immediate aftermath of a stressful event, adrenaline secretion increases.

What does all this mean? When GABA is not inhibiting the other neurotransmitters, they become more active, which causes a stimulating effect. The increased stimulation of serotonin and dopamine (not being inhibited by GABA) can increase the possibility of developing depression or anxiety. With an increase of dopamine, we are more likely to experience negative thinking and racing thoughts. This is when we are more likely to escalate the effect of a minor issue—in other words, make a mountain out of a molehill. Symptoms are worsened by the secretion of adrenaline, which excites the brain and body, and our chances of rational thinking decrease even more.

SELF-REFLECTION

Think about a situation in which you experienced anxiety. Do you remember how you reacted? Were you confused or frightened by the feeling? What, if any, were the physical symptoms? Write down what you remember about the situation.

The Anxiety Checklist

This checklist will help determine the type of anxiety you are experiencing. Place a checkmark beside all statements that describe you.

Category A

- ☐ I have an intense fear of a specific object/situation (e.g., snakes, heights).
- ☐ I almost always feel afraid when facing this object/situation.
- ☐ I try to avoid this object/situation; if I must face it, I feel intensely afraid.
- ☐ My fear seems out of proportion to the actual danger.
- ☐ I've had this fear for many months.
- ☐ This fear causes problems in my daily life.

Category B

- ☐ I have intense fear or anxiety about social/performance situations (e.g., meeting new people, giving a speech).
- ☐ In these situations, I'm afraid I will show anxiety (i.e., blushing or trembling) and people will think less of me.
- ☐ I'm nearly always anxious or afraid in these situations.
- ☐ I try to avoid these situations or face them with intense fear.
- ☐ My fear seems too great for the actual threat in the situation.
- ☐ I've feared or avoided these situations for many months.
- ☐ This fear or avoidance creates problems in my daily life.

Category C

- ☐ I've experienced sudden episodes of intense and overwhelming fear that seemed to come out of the blue.

- [ ] During these episodes, I experienced four or more of the following symptoms: racing or pounding heart, sweating, shaking, breathlessness, choking sensations, chest pain or discomfort, nausea or stomachache, dizziness or faintness, chills or feeling hot, numbness or tingling, feeling of unreality or detachment, feelings of loss of control or "going crazy," or feeling afraid to die.

- [ ] I worry about having more episodes and try to avoid them (e.g., by avoiding exercise that might raise my heart rate or cause shortness of breath).

Category D

- [ ] I have intense fear of at least two of the following: public transportation, open spaces, enclosed spaces, standing in line or in a crowd, or going out of my home alone.

- [ ] I fear or avoid these situations because it would be hard to escape or get help if I had a panic attack or emergency.

- [ ] These situations nearly always make me afraid.

- [ ] I avoid these situations or endure them with much anxiety.

- [ ] My fear seems out of proportion to the actual danger involved.

- [ ] I've feared these situations for many months.

- [ ] This fear causes problems in my daily life.

Category E

- [ ] I worry excessively about many things most days (e.g., job responsibilities, health, finances).

- [ ] I find it hard to control my worry.

- [ ] I've worried like this for several months.

- [ ] When I worry, I've experienced at least a few of the following symptoms: restlessness, being easily tired, difficulty thinking, irritability, muscle tension, or trouble sleeping.

- [ ] These worries cause problems in my daily life.

Each category corresponds to a specific anxiety disorder. Check if your symptoms fall mostly in one or more of the following categories.

- ❏   A: Specific phobia
- ❏   B. Social anxiety disorder
- ❏   C: Panic disorder
- ❏   D: Agoraphobia
- ❏   E: Generalized anxiety disorder

Talk to Your Doctor

Attention! If you think you have an undiagnosed anxiety disorder or have been experiencing long-term, chronic insomnia and are having mental/physical issues as a result, please meet with your doctor or seek emergency services.

CHANGE YOUR BRAIN, CHANGE YOUR SLEEP

Our brains have the capacity for change. The technical term for this ability is neuroplasticity. I like to think about the chemical responses in our brain as a pathway on a map. If you take the same route on a map (or through the brain), the pathway gets larger or deeper. These are the tracks that we have traveled frequently. Fortunately, as with a map, there are alternate routes in the brain, and we can change the ones we take.

Cognitive behavioral therapy (CBT) is ideal for changing the pathways in our brain because it helps us change our response to stress. Change happens consciously at first, and with repeated use of CBT tools, you will begin to unconsciously use those techniques and hopefully reduce anxiety levels and sleep better. Often, our learned sleep habits can interfere with our ability to get to sleep or stay asleep. Learning how to change these detrimental sleep habits and what can be reasonably expected of sleep can help you modify your thinking about rest and help you get to sleep more easily.

With less anxiety and easier sleep, you will have more energy to do the things that really matter to you. You'll likely find life more pleasant and find it much easier to reach any goals you have set. As the negativity associated with anxiety reduces, you will become more positive about life.

CBT begins with setting a goal. When you have a goal (no more than two nights of poor sleep per month, for example), you've already set a path toward recovery because you now know which tools will work best for you on your path to avoiding insomnia. Once you begin to use the tools of CBT, your behavior will change how you think about your stress issues by changing how you feel. For instance, in my clinic, I see many shorter-than-average sleepers who are spending too much time in bed. When I tell them they will have to change their behavior consistently for two weeks for the brain to change its patterns, they are often skeptical. But when I see them at their first follow-up appointment three to four weeks later, their demeanor is much more positive and hopeful. This is what changing your behavior and changing those pathways in your brain can do for you.

CBT can be a successful treatment for insomnia and anxiety because it boosts your confidence and belief that you are capable of making positive changes in your life. You change your behavior, which is something that you can control. Medications can help with insomnia and anxiety, but they sometimes have undesirable side effects. In addition, medications often lose their effectiveness after a period of time because your body can adapt to the chemicals, and they can also produce psychological dependence. The pill becomes the stimulus to maintain balance rather than your desire to be well. Therefore, behavioral modification makes more sense. The more you practice, the better you get at making changes and seeing what works for you, and, most importantly, the better you feel.

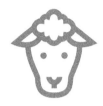

REVIEW & REFLECT

You've learned about the science behind anxiety and insomnia, and you likely have a better sense about what causes it and its effects on your mind and body. Using the space provided below and on the next page, think about your anxiety, your insomnia, and what motivates you to overcome it. What aspects of your life are you looking to improve?

_____

_____

_____

_____

_____

MOVING FORWARD

In this chapter, we've learned about the benefits of adequate sleep. We have also learned how a lack of sleep can affect our body and cognition. A lack of sleep causes stress and can worsen anxiety and depressive symptoms. You also are realizing that there are many people that have similar symptoms, so you are not alone.

In addition, we have learned that with the help of CBT, it is possible to change how we think and, therefore, how we respond to our anxiety symptoms.

In the next section, we will learn more about CBT and the tools and techniques used to change the tracks in our brain.

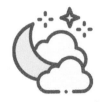

CHAPTER TWO

The Gold Standard

· ·

In this chapter, we will be discussing CBT and CBT-I. These two therapies are considered the gold standard for treatment of anxiety and insomnia, respectively, because they have the longest-lasting effects. CBT and CBT-I help people make behavioral changes in their lives, altering habits that contribute to anxiety and insomnia. You will learn about medications and substances used for insomnia and anxiety, and I will also provide you with some other tools to guide you through the tough spots as you change your behavior.

THE POWER OF CBT

CBT tools have been used to help people with anxiety and depression for many years with a great deal of success. In the 1950s, Dr. Albert Ellis proposed rational emotive behavior therapy (REBT), which focused on behavioral and emotional problems. In the 1960s, Dr. Aaron Beck began treating his patients with cognitive therapy, helping them recognize negative, self-sabotaging thoughts, and teaching them to redirect their thinking to alleviate symptoms. Dr. Beck's therapy focused mainly on cognition—in other words, the ability to acquire and understand knowledge and then apply it to your life. The introduction of CBT techniques for the treatment of insomnia and depression is attributed to both of these theorists/practitioners. By combining CBT and REBT, we cover the cognitive, behavioral, and emotional components of anxiety and insomnia. It is the gold standard because it has been effective for up to 80 percent of compliant patients, according to *Simply Psychology*.

Before setting a goal for therapy, make a list of your strengths. If you're unsure, ask friends or family what they feel are your strengths. This will help you stay positive as you set your goal.

A goal will give you a vision of the future and make committing to the therapy much easier. When choosing a goal, there are several things you will want to keep in mind. Keep it realistic, simple, and achievable, and choose one that is important to you—you'll more likely be able to meet it that way. As you change your behavior and gain confidence in your ability to apply CBT techniques, you can increase your goal's complexity and degree of challenge.

It's also a good idea to journal about your progress and document your pathway. This does two things for you: First, it gives you a written account about how far you have progressed with your goal. Second, it provides you with a road map to which you can return, if necessary, at some future date.

There are several techniques that CBT uses to help you reach your goal, and we will cover them more fully in later chapters.

Relaxation

Intentional relaxation entails a specific process. Sit quietly in a comfortable position—one in which you will not fall asleep. Close your eyes and feel the weight of your body sink into the seat, allowing your limbs to become heavy. Remain relaxed and begin counting each breath. Do this for 20 minutes, but don't set an alarm; only open your eyes to check the time. Remain passive, and if distracting thoughts occur, ignore them and keep counting.

Coping

Coping deals with fear. When anxiety is triggered, the first thoughts tend to be the worst-case scenario. Identify your deepest fear and write down a detailed description of the scenario. Imagine how this tragedy would affect your health, your family and relationships, your work and education, your home obligations, and how you spend your leisure time. How would it alter the meaning of your life? What will your quality of life be like? How will you cope? Review this scenario over several days. Try to become as emotionally involved in the scenario as possible. Over time, you will notice a decrease in your anxiety as you put yourself into the scenario. When your anxiety is reduced by 50 percent, begin working on a plan for how you will cope with this issue; use the same sheet of paper on which you described the scenario of your fear. For the next two weeks, take time in your day to imagine how you will successfully cope with the issue.

Resilience

Building resilience is one of the keys to successful CBT. Resilient people view problems as predictable and controllable. They believe that what they do is important—which increases their confidence and commitment to their work—and that they have control over many of life's events. A sense of control reduces the impact of the stressor. The person realizes that if they don't have control, they need to release it because it's not worth their energy. They also see problems as challenges, which is a more positive view of the issue. Resilience is correlated with happiness (it's hard to be happy and stressed at the same time). Retrain your brain to be resilient by asking yourself if you have any control over the situation. If not, let it go. If so, change it. Try to reframe your issues as challenges rather than problems.

Stress Management

Several stress-management techniques are helpful for dealing with anxiety. One of these is managing expectations. If you're able to avoid projecting expectations on an outcome and simply accept what occurs, you're less likely to be anxious when the outcome doesn't happen as you had planned. Developing an exercise plan has also been shown to reduce anxiety, as has diaphragmatic breathing. But probably the most important thing you can do is challenge automatic thoughts. Writing down unwanted thoughts will help you identify how your thinking may be misguided.

Assertiveness

Assertiveness is helpful for anxiety-prone individuals. Letting others know what you think about an issue often feels prohibitive. But learning to express your ideas in a clear and direct way can help alleviate anxiety by putting you in control and allowing self-expression. When you don't express your thoughts, anxiety can worsen because you are keeping those thoughts and ideas bottled up.

Success with CBT

Recent studies show that self-guided CBT is as effective as counselor-guided CBT, but these results need to be read with caution as there is a significant difference in CBT materials with each study. As noted previously, counselor-guided cognitive therapy has an effectiveness of about 80 percent. Despite this, for certain motivated people, self-guided CBT is a very good place to begin treatment.

TRANSFORMATION THROUGH CBT-I ···········

CBT-I was adopted by sleep physicians long before psychologists became interested in treating insomnia. In his 1999 book, *The Promise of Sleep*, William Dement writes about his nearly 50 years of research in sleep. In his chapter on insomnia, he refers to sleep hygiene, relaxation, stimulus control, cognitive techniques, and sleep restriction. CBT-I applies the theory of CBT to those experiencing insomnia—helping them transform their thinking patterns—and adds other techniques unique to sleep to help people get to sleep much faster and stay asleep more easily.

The cognitive part of CBT-I has to do with rethinking sleep. The first task is to determine your sleep need, which is different for everyone. We determine sleep need by keeping a sleep log (see page 53 for sleep log examples). These logs provide you with information about your sleep patterns and the quantity of sleep you need. Your body will sleep when it needs to sleep. So sleep can occur at inopportune times—like while driving or performing other tasks requiring alertness—if you're not proactive about sleep. When you've completed your sleep log, your sleep need can be calculated as an average. You'll then begin sleep-period restriction, which is simply restricting your time in bed.

In general, your average sleep time plus 30 to 60 minutes is all the time you should be spending in bed. It takes about two weeks of maintaining a consistent schedule for your brain to begin to adjust to a new sleep period, so persistence is important. Once you get past the first two weeks, you should start to feel better, and the improvement will likely continue with time.

Stimulus Control

Stimulus control simply means controlling the stimuli in your environment to invite sleep. There are several things that you can do to optimize your sleep. For instance, light wakes us up, so dimming lights in the evening and getting plenty of light on your face in the morning is important to help you fall asleep and wake up. In the light spectrum, it is the blue ray that hits the photoreceptors in our eyes to wake us up. Computer and smartphone screens are backed by blue light and were meant to keep us awake, so screens are not an issue in the morning but should be turned off one hour prior to bedtime. Eating within four hours of bedtime raises your metabolic rate and warms the body core, which can make sleep difficult. Exercising within four to five hours of bedtime also energizes you. It's not a good idea to go to bed if you aren't sleepy because you may have difficulty getting to sleep. That, then, increases the likelihood of becoming frustrated about your inability to sleep, which arouses emotion and makes it even more difficult to get to sleep. Removing the emotional arousal around sleep is extremely important.

Substances

Substances—including tobacco, alcohol, and caffeine—can interfere with the ability to sleep. I generally advise individuals to avoid caffeine within eight hours of bedtime. Though you may be able to get to sleep after drinking caffeine, the stimulation of the brain keeps you in the lighter stages of sleep. Alcohol may facilitate sleep, but when metabolized by the liver about four hours after going to sleep, it can wake you up or, at least, bump you into the shallower stages of sleep. Tobacco acts as a stimulant, so I generally recommend no tobacco within four hours of bedtime.

Biological Clock

The body regulates sleep through the use of the biological clock and the sleep/wake homeostasis mechanism, which is the balance of sleep and wakefulness. These two systems interact to make sleep relatively different from person to person. The biological clock determines the timing of sleep, so one person may find it easy and comfortable to wake early in the morning and go to bed relatively early in the evening. By contrast, another may prefer to stay awake until the wee hours of the morning and have difficulty getting out of bed the following day. The biological clock does not always respond to social cues easily, and treatment to reset it may be required. In other words, there are ways to shift your biological clock.

Regulation of the Sleep Schedule

Finally, being attentive to your body's natural need for stability and regulation is important. Eating breakfast is important for those with insomnia because it cues the body to awaken and provides energy for the day. A good way to prepare your body for sleep is to develop a nighttime routine where you make sure to complete any busy activities at least 30 minutes prior to bedtime, and then spend that time doing something calming and relaxing. This could be listening to calming music, meditating, praying, progressive muscle relaxation (see page 35), coloring, doing word puzzles, or reading (reading material should be interesting, but something that can be set aside at any time). Developing these habits can improve the quality of your sleep.

Complementary Therapy: ACT

Acceptance and commitment therapy (ACT) is a method for reframing how you think about problematic issues in your life. Individuals build their mental flexibility by learning to accept those issues that are out of their control. In addition, ACT uses mindfulness (see page 36) to reduce racing thoughts and assist with staying in the moment. This therapy can be effective in dealing with moderate to severe anxiety or depression. It can also be very effective for individuals who have problems turning off their thoughts at bedtime and for those who need help recognizing and accepting (not denying) their sleep problems. In ACT, individuals learn to "go with" the feeling/problem (a form of acceptance) rather than catastrophizing it. When emotions get involved with a problem, it becomes very hard to release the issue; for an individual with insomnia who is likely sleep deprived, it becomes monumentally harder. Avoiding emotional entanglement allows sleep to come more easily. In addition, ACT helps individuals analyze cognitive distortions, which allows for identification of negative thought pathways and reframing of thought patterns.

SELF-REFLECTION

Are you familiar with CBT or CBT-I? What do you hope to achieve from using CBT and CBT-I to combat your anxiety and insomnia?

_____

_____

_____

_____

_____

SLEEP AIDS ··

This book takes a drug-free approach but acknowledges that, in some cases, medication or supplements may be necessary. Prescription sleep aids were originally meant to be used only temporarily for those stressful life situations in which sleep is interrupted. Habitual use of any type of sleep aid does not provide you with healthy sleep. Some of these substances are psychologically addictive. In my work with sleep patients, I do more to get people off of sleep aids than to prescribe them.

While we cannot recommend sleep aids (anything you take should be either prescribed or recommended by your medical provider), the following are a few of the most often used aids. Make sure you have a full understanding of how these may interfere with any other medication you take and how they may affect you overall.

Prescriptions

Most prescription hypnotics are controlled substances that have addictive potential. One of the most commonly used drugs is Ambien (zolpidem), which is used for getting to sleep and treating sleep-onset insomnia. Ambien CR is used for staying asleep and treating sleep-maintenance insomnia. You need to be in bed for about seven hours if you take Ambien or roughly eight hours with Ambien CR. Side effects include abnormal sleep behavior—such as sleep walking and sleep talking—nightmares, and sleep inertia (a sort of hungover effect from the drug). Ambien has been reported to cause memory problems as well. Another commonly used sleep medication is Lunesta (eszopiclone), which is used for sleep-maintenance problems. Like Ambien, you should spend seven hours in bed when you take it, and the pill should not be broken in half. The most common side effect is a metallic taste, and it can also cause headaches and sleep inertia the following day.

Benzodiazepines treat both anxiety and sleep problems; unfortunately, they can be highly addictive. The one most commonly used for sleep is temazepam, which is primarily used for sleep-onset problems, but it can also be used for sleep-maintenance insomnia. Common side effects of this medication include sleep inertia, headache, and lightheadedness. If you have been on benzodiazepines for more than a few months, you'll need to wean yourself off the medication slowly to avoid negative side effects.

Serotonin modulators were originally formulated to treat anxiety and depression, but one in particular, trazodone, is commonly used for sleep maintenance. Trazodone has very few side effects—the main one being sleep inertia—but it does not work for everyone. Its use for sleep is off-label; in other words, it has not been FDA-approved to use for sleep, but it is used frequently despite this.

Over-the-Counter (OTC) Sleep Aids

Over-the-counter (OTC) sleep aids contain antihistamines and sometimes supplements. The most commonly used OTC sleep aid is Benadryl (diphenhydramine). It has the effect of putting you to sleep, but it often causes sleep inertia upon awakening. Tylenol PM and Advil PM are a combination of a pain reliever and diphenhydramine, and they have the same side effects as Benadryl. Diphenhydramine is the only ingredient in Simply Sleep; NyQuil, however, is a little different and is used to help with nighttime colds and coughs. It contains acetaminophen for pain and fever, dextromethorphan to suppress cough, and doxylamine succinate for allergy issues and sleep. Its newer sister, ZzzQuil, is another formulation of diphenhydramine.

Supplements

Melatonin is one of the most commonly used supplements for sleep. It is a similar substance to the melatonin that is produced by the brain to promote sleep and comes in various formulations and dosages. The time-release form can help with sleep maintenance, while the immediate-release form is best for sleep-onset issues. Timing your melatonin dose can be tricky, and it can vary depending on the type of sleep issue you are experiencing. Side effects of melatonin include vivid, odd dreams and sleep inertia.

GABA is a supplement that is also used for sleep. It is similar to the neurotransmitter GABA produced in the brain and is thought to calm the brain and help induce and maintain sleep. It is also thought to reduce anxiety. It does react with many medications, so consult your doctor before taking GABA if you are on other medications or supplements. Side effects are primarily gastrointestinal and include nausea and loss of appetite.

Valerian root is an herb that has been used for many years for sleep and in the treatment of anxiety and depression. It is believed to improve sleep quality, but it may not help you get to sleep. Lavender is a plant that has a pleasant, calming scent and has been used for sleep as well. In addition, chamomile tea is thought to have calming properties that help people get to sleep.

Magnesium is a mineral that is thought to calm the brain and nervous system, thereby inducing sleep.

SELF-REFLECTION

Have you tried sleep aids? What has your experience been with them? Were they positive? Were they negative? Which worked for you?

_____

_____

_____

_____

_____

RELAXATION AND ALTERNATIVE METHODS · · · · ·

Beyond CBT-I, other approaches may work to calm the mind and body and aid sleep. These can be useful for comorbid insomnia as well as those who do shift work or frequently experience jet lag. They are all techniques that help shift your focus to your body or thought processes.

Progressive Muscle Relaxation

This technique is helpful for pain and relaxation and takes the relaxation technique of CBT one step further. While counting your breath, contract and relax one muscle group at a time from your toes to your face. Continue counting your breath after you have contracted and released all large muscle groups. This technique takes the tension out of the muscles and allows for full relaxation. It also helps you relax your mind and focus on your body.

Meditation

Meditation helps with focus because it literally asks you to focus on an object or how you are feeling in some part of your body and to monitor your thoughts. When I meditate, I like to have a bouquet of helium balloons in my mind's eye. I imagine myself attaching an intrusive thought to each balloon, and then watch it float away into the clouds. Meditation clears the mind of unwanted thoughts by allowing them to pass by without paying attention to or following them. It teaches the mind discipline, and, when you're good at it, you will find that you have fewer intrusive thoughts when you're not meditating because you've trained your brain to avoid giving any attention to unwanted thoughts.

Mindfulness

When we're performing activities that don't require focus, our minds tend to wander either to reviewing past events or anticipating future events. In addition, our minds also tend to evaluate our current circumstances in a binary fashion—our current reality is either good or bad based on whether outcomes are favorable for us. Mindfulness requires focus on the current situation so that you can fully appreciate what's going on around you. This benefits you in two ways: First, you're getting more out of the current reality, and, second, you avoid the intrusive thoughts that occur when you allow your mind to wander.

External Tools

Light is an important part of the sleep cycle, and it can be used to our benefit. Getting plenty of light on your face upon awakening will help you become alert in the morning. Likewise, dimming light in the evening before bedtime can help usher in sleep. Temperature is important as well. To get to sleep, our core body temperature decreases, so taking a hot shower prior to bedtime can help some people get to sleep more easily by dilating surface blood vessels to release heat. Also, keeping the temperature in your bedroom cooler helps maintain sleep. White or pink noise can also reduce intrusive thoughts and give your brain something else to focus on. White and pink noise can be found on smartphone apps.

Laughter Therapy

Laughter therapy has been found to help the elderly improve the quality of their sleep and helps them get to sleep and stay asleep more easily. Developing a sense of humor and being able to laugh at life circumstances has been shown to ward off negative thinking. It also alleviates stress, depression, anxiety, and insomnia. If you have a hard time laughing and developing a sense of humor, enlist the help of family and friends.

SELF-REFLECTION

Take a closer look at these relaxation and alternative methods. Are you familiar with these methods? Which do you feel comfortable using?

_____

_____

_____

_____

_____

_____

SITTING WITH UNEASINESS ·······················

When we're dealing with uncomfortable issues, we often forget that our body is designed to protect us from perceived danger. The brain is constantly making predictions about our future based on past experience. These predictions are then used to direct our future. Anxiety and uneasiness occur when we fail to make appropriate predictions based on our past experience. It can be extremely difficult to manage our thoughts when we're feeling anxious. There are several things we can do to make "sitting with uneasiness" bearable.

We learned in chapter 1 how our bodies respond to anxiety. When we become aware of bodily responses, we can intervene and change how our bodies respond to a stressor. For instance, if your heart is racing and your breathing quickens, it may help to take several deep, cleansing breaths to reduce your heart rate and slow your breathing. A reduction in the body's response to anxiety can help reduce your emotional response as well.

Another way to cope with uneasiness is to confront your fears with a reality check. For instance, let's say you've been asked to give a speech in front of an audience on a topic that you know very well. Despite being an expert on the topic, you fear being in front of a large group of people. In that case, you may benefit from focusing on the fact that you're the expert in the room and that most audience members will know much less than you do about the topic. This will hopefully reassure you and give you confidence.

Mindfulness (see page 36) is another excellent way to manage uneasiness because it keeps us in the moment. We remain focused on what's going on in the present moment rather than concerning ourselves with past problems or future unknowns. Often, if we can consistently stay in the moment, we find that there's a lot to learn and experience. Many people find a great deal of joy and peace when they stay in the moment, and it also helps us simply slow down a bit.

We often try to get as many tasks completed as we can, but underestimating the amount of time it takes to complete a task can cause anxiety. On the other hand, if we allow ourselves a buffer between tasks that we need to complete, we will be less likely to awaken anxious thoughts.

Sometimes, recognizing the patterns of uneasiness may help you preempt anxiety. If you realize that you get anxious at bedtime because you anticipate the tasks you have before you when you wake up, you may benefit from preparing for your next day by having some things ready the night before. Perhaps you can pack your lunch and lay out your clothes for the next day. In addition, a bedtime routine is a good way to reduce uneasiness and usher in a good night's sleep.

When you're able to sleep well, memory is consolidated. Energy levels increase, and you have more stamina than you would with poor sleep. Getting adequate sleep decreases our anxiety levels and increases our ability to learn new things.

It is important to remember that your sleep patterns, schedule, and the amount of sleep you require are unique to you. For instance, some individuals can sleep anywhere, whereas others need everything in their environment to be just right in order to get to sleep. Learn your sensitivities and be sure your environment is conducive to sleep.

Reward System

Develop a system for rewarding yourself when you reach certain points in your treatment. Make your reward something that's important to you and that you're willing to work hard for so that it motivates you to maintain your program. Since we already know that coping with anxiety and insomnia are difficult and time consuming, a reward system may encourage you to continue until you get the desired results.

One Size Does Not Fit All

The traditional 9 a.m. to 5 p.m. work schedule does not fit all employment situations. Nor does the standard 10 p.m. bedtime and 6 a.m. wake time. Feel free to be creative and thoughtful about what you really wish to change about your sleep habits; there's more than one way to accomplish your goals. For instance, if you go to bed at 2 a.m. and wake up at 10 a.m., and it fits into your work schedule and lifestyle, you may not need to change your sleep schedule at all.

Journaling

I cannot overstate the importance of journaling throughout this process. Over time, and as you find success, you will want to look back on your progress and give yourself a pat on the back for a job well done. Sometimes, especially if we get positive results from the changes we make, we forget where we began. It's good to remind yourself of your progress, which reinforces the positive feelings you get from your success. It also gives you a track record of how you were able to strategize your changes in the event of a setback.

SELF-REFLECTION

Are you ready to commit to dealing with discomfort? Acknowledge that this process is likely to be difficult and may bring up uneasy feelings for you. But also, think about the reasons you've decided to start this workbook and what you're working toward.

_____

_____

_____

_____

_____

_____

_____

MOVING FORWARD ·

In this chapter, we learned that CBT is a goal-oriented treatment for both insomnia and anxiety. We begin by setting small, achievable goals that are important to us. We also learned that CBT-I is the gold standard for treating insomnia and that rethinking our sleep starts with determining how much sleep we need. We reviewed several sleep aids, including common prescriptions and over-the-counter medications, and discussed several alternative methods to help induce sleep.

In the next chapter, you will assess your sleep need, do a sleep self-assessment, complete sleep diaries, and calculate your sleep need. You will also assess the severity of your insomnia. Finally, you will set a goal for achieving better sleep.

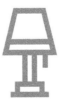

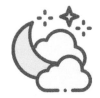

CHAPTER THREE

Baseline & Sleep Assessment

. . . .

This chapter will lead you through the assessment of your sleep. By the end, you should have some idea about the changes you could consider to improve your sleep habits. You will be introduced to the sleep logs (also known as sleep diaries), which are probably the most important part of this exercise because they will show you patterns in your sleep and sleep habits. They will also help you set your goals for obtaining a restful night's sleep.

HOW MUCH SLEEP DO YOU NEED? ··············

The latest research done by the National Sleep Foundation recommends that adults aged 18 to 64 get seven to nine hours of sleep per night and that adults aged 65 and older should obtain seven to eight hours of sleep per night. However, this "recommendation" only applies to about 65 percent of the population. The sleep needs of the remainder of the population are typically outside these boundaries.

Every person has a different need for sleep. Some can get by on as little as four hours of sleep, while others need up to 14 hours of sleep per day. It's important to know how much sleep you need so that you can plan for it. Being proactive about sleep is extremely important because, as we have already learned, adequate sleep will help us stay healthier.

Did your difficulty with sleep begin suddenly, or have you had difficulty getting to sleep or staying asleep most of your life? If your symptoms started suddenly, can you pinpoint when they began? If so, think about what was going on in your life. Were you experiencing a change in employment or in one of your relationships? Was there a death in the family, a personal crisis, or a new medical or mental illness diagnosis? Often, we get into the habit of sleeping poorly because we're under stress, and, when the stressor resolves, we forget to resume our healthier sleep habits.

If you've had difficulty with sleep much of your life, think about how you have slept in the past. Can you remember a season when you slept well and woke up feeling refreshed and energetic for a two- to three-month period of time? Do you recall how many hours of sleep you were getting at that time? Ask a parent if you were a good or poor sleeper as a baby, or if you were a longer- or shorter-than-normal sleeper as a baby. Were you a good napper as a toddler? As a child, if you participated in childhood sleepovers with peers, were you the first to go to sleep or the last? Were you the first to wake up or the last? Generally, if we were short sleepers as children, we will be short sleepers as adults. Similarly, if we were long sleepers as children, we may need more time in bed than normal as adults.

If there was ever a season when sleep came easily to you, think about how long you were spending in bed at the time. If you are retired, how much sleep did you get when you were working? Perhaps that schedule could be resumed if you are having difficulty now. Were you in the military? The amount of sleep you got while serving may give you a clue about your sleep need.

When you go on vacation, how much sleep do you get? Often, vacations are packed with activities, and we are relaxed and under less stress. In that context, we often find it easier to sleep.

Sometimes, it is difficult to determine your sleep need even after answering these questions. In that case, using a sleep log will help you determine where to start with restricting your sleep period.

We will begin with the sleep self-assessment, which you will find on the next page.

The Sleep Self-Assessment

Sometimes, the patterns in our lives are not ideal for helping us get to sleep or stay asleep. This assessment will help you pinpoint the habits that may be impairing your sleep and set goals for better sleep later.

Answer the following questions to determine what your sleep and sleep habits have been like for the past month.

1. What time did you go to bed? If it varies, provide a range of times. _____

2. Is your bedroom cool, quiet, dark, and comfortable? _____

3. How long did it take you to fall asleep? If it varies, provide a range of times. _____

4. How many times did you wake up in the night? Did you get out of bed each time? _____

5. How long did it take you to return to sleep? If it varies, provide a range of times. _____

6. What time did you wake up? If it varies, provide a range of times. _____

7. On a scale of 1 to 10 (where 1 is extremely sleepy and 10 is fully rested), how did you feel on awakening in the morning on most days? _____

8. Did you take a sleeping pill or an over-the-counter sleep aid to get to sleep? _____

9. Did you drink caffeinated beverages to stay energized during the day? If so, did you drink them within eight hours of bedtime? _____

10. Did you drink alcohol within four hours of bedtime? _____

11. Do you do anything in bed other than sleep or activities relating to intimacy or sickness? _____

12. Do you turn off screens one hour before bedtime? _____

13. Do you engage in a nightly bedtime routine to prepare your body for sleep?

    _____

14. Do you feel like your mind races at bedtime or when you wake in the night, making it difficult to return to sleep? _____

15. Do you watch the clock in the night? If so, do you find yourself calculating how much time you have left to sleep until your scheduled wake time? _____

16. Do you get anxious or frustrated because you cannot return to sleep? _____

17. Do you nap? If so, how long are your naps, and what time of day do you typically nap? _____

18. Does pain or stress interfere with your ability to get to sleep or stay asleep? _____

19. Do you have environmental factors that interfere with sleep (i.e. children, pets, being on call for work, noisy neighbors)? _____

20. Do you feel the need to cancel planned activities due to sleepiness or fatigue? _____

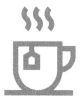

SELF-REFLECTION

Think about the last time you slept well, woke up the next morning feeling refreshed, and had energy during the day. How many hours did you sleep? What were your sleep conditions? What did your life look like? What does an ideal night's sleep look like for you? How many hours of sleep would you like to get each night?

_____

_____

_____

_____

_____

_____

_____

_____

_____

_____

_____

_____

_____

_____

_____

_____

_____

_____

_____

_____

_____

_____

_____

_____

_____

_____

_____

_____

_____

_____

_____

_____

_____

_____

_____

_____

The Insomnia Severity Assessment

This assessment measures how being sleepy or tired is affecting your daily life and ability to function. Each question should be answered with a number from 1 to 4, as shown below, to describe the difficulty you have with each task as a result of sleepiness or tiredness. Place N/A in the blank if the question does not apply to you.

1 – YES, EXTREME DIFFICULTY

2 – YES, MODERATE DIFFICULTY

3 – YES, A LITTLE DIFFICULTY

4 – NO DIFFICULTY

1. Do you have difficulty concentrating on the things you do because you are sleepy or tired? _____

2. Do you have difficulty remembering things because you are sleepy or tired? _____

3. Do you have difficulty working on a hobby because you are sleepy or tired? _____

4. Do you have difficulty doing housework because you are sleepy or tired? _____

5. Do you have difficulty operating a motor vehicle for *short* distances (fewer than 100 miles) because you are sleepy or tired? _____

6. Do you have difficulty operating a motor vehicle for *long* distances (more than 100 miles) because you are sleepy or tired? _____

7. Do you have difficulty getting things done because you are too tired or sleepy to drive or take public transportation? _____

8. Do you have difficulty taking care of financial affairs and doing paperwork because you are sleepy or tired? _____

9. Do you have difficulty performing employed or volunteer work because you are too sleepy or tired? _____

10. Do you have difficulty visiting with your family or friends in *their* homes because you become sleepy or tired? _____

11. Do you have difficulty doing things for your family or friends because you are too sleepy or tired? _____

12. Has your relationship with family, friends, or work colleagues been affected because you are sleepy or tired? _____

13. Do you have difficulty exercising or participating in a sporting activity because you are too sleepy or tired? _____

14. Do you have difficulty watching a movie or video because you become sleepy or tired? _____

15. Do you have difficulty watching TV because you are sleepy or tired? _____

16. Do you have difficulty being as active as you want in the *evening* because you are too sleepy or tired? _____

17. Do you have difficulty being as active as you want in the *morning* because you are too sleepy or tired? _____

18. Do you have difficulty being as active as you want in the *afternoon* because you are too sleepy or tired? _____

19. Has your intimate or sexual relationship been affected because you are sleepy or tired? _____

20. Has your desire for intimacy or sex been affected because you are sleepy or tired? _____

To calculate your score, simply add up your answers and divide by the number of questions you answered. This will give you a number between 1 and 4. The result can be read as follows:

0 to 1.5 – Extreme dysfunction

1.6 to 2.5 – Moderate dysfunction

2.6 to 3.5 – Mild dysfunction

3.6 to 4 – No dysfunction

(Adapted from FOSQ, Weaver, 1997)

Determining Your Sleep Drive

The body's sleep drive balances wakefulness and sleep. Over the course of a day, the longer we are awake, the stronger our sleep drive becomes. If we have a regular sleep schedule, our sleep drive becomes intense at about the same time every day. A strong sleep drive makes it easier to get to sleep and stay asleep. If the sleep drive were the only mechanism that regulates our sleep, it would make sense that we are more alert in the morning and more tired in the evening. But it's not the only mechanism that controls our sleep cycle. Our sleep drive is affected by our biological clock, which deals with the timing of sleep that is unique to each one of us. If you are naturally a morning person, your sleep drive likely peaks in the early to mid-evening. If you are a night owl, your sleep drive will more likely peak in the later evening or early morning. If you are neither, your sleep drive will likely peak somewhere between the two.

THE SLEEP LOG

The sleep log (or diary) is a record of your sleep, wakefulness, and habits around sleep, and it also measures your daytime sleepiness and fatigue. A sleep log can help you track your sleep patterns and give you a baseline from which to begin to change your sleep habits. Ideally, you should track your sleep for at least two weeks to one month. This will give you an idea about how your sleep patterns change on a day-to-day basis.

When you wake up in the morning, take about five minutes to complete the part of the sleep log relating to the night before. The sleep log should include the date and bedtime (the time that you actually turned out the lights to attempt sleep). Next, log how long it took you to get to sleep. If this part of the sleep log causes you to watch the clock, turn the clock away from you; you don't need to know what time it is during the night. Watching the clock can stimulate racing thoughts or cause you to do "nighttime math"—calculating how many more hours you have left to sleep—which typically worsens insomnia. Instead, to get a sense for what 15 minutes feels like when

Sleep Log

Complete this Section After Getting Out of Bed | Complete at End of Day

Day and date	Unusual stressors: time of Alcohol & sleep medication	Time you went to bed	Time it took you to fall asleep	# of awakenings	Amount of time awake	Time you got up for the day	Total sleep time	Sleepiness Rating (see below)	Fatigue Rating	Napping: time of day & sleep amount

*Amount of time awake: this is all the time you spent awake during the night, from the first time you awakened to the time you got out of bed. It does not include the time it took you to fall asleep initially.

Sleepiness and Fatigue Rating Scale: (Average Rating for the Whole Day Following A Given Sleep Episode)

	0	25	50	75	100
SLEEPINESS:	Extremely Sleepy	Sleepy	Neither	Alert	Very Alert
FATIGUE:	Extremely Fatigued	Fatigued	Neither	Energetic	Very Energetic

you're in bed waiting for sleep to arrive, time yourself during the day doing nothing for 15 minutes (make sure you use a timer). This will give you an idea of what 15 minutes feels like when you're idle.

Next, note the number of times you woke up and the total amount of time you were awake. Calculate the estimated amount of time you were in bed and subtract from that the amount of time you were awake (how long it took you to get to sleep, plus the total time you were awake in the middle of the night) to get your total sleep time. Make sure to list any stressors you experienced prior to sleep. If anything in particular awakened you—pain, a pet, a bedpartner, etc.—note it in the log. In addition, if you took something to get to sleep, that information may also be helpful. List any activities that you did (other than sleep and intimacy) in bed. All of this information will aid in the analysis of your sleep log.

The last part of the log is about your day. Think about your entire day, not just how you feel at bedtime. Then, before going to bed, answer the following three questions: First, rate your sleepiness on a scale of 1 to 100 (where 1 is extremely sleepy and 100 is very alert). Second, rate your fatigue on a scale of 1 to 100 (where 1 is extremely fatigued and 100 is very energetic). Last, if you took a nap, note the time you napped and how long you slept.

You are looking for patterns in your sleep. For instance, if you spent extra time in bed on the weekend, did you notice that it was harder to get to sleep on Sunday night? If this is the case, regulating your wake time (getting up at the same time every day) may be helpful. Do you notice that you spend a few days getting a lot of sleep (nine to 10 hours) followed by a few days of very little sleep (four to five hours)? This variability could indicate that you are oversleeping on some days and not getting enough sleep on others.

If you were unable to determine your sleep need from the self-assessment, use the information recorded in your sleep log. It is simply an average of your total sleep time. Add the total sleep hours of every day you've recorded, and divide that sum by the number of days you recorded a total sleep time. Then, restrict your time in bed to that time plus 30 to 60 minutes. Remember, it takes about two weeks of a relatively rigid sleep schedule to train your brain to sleep when you want; it may take up to two weeks before you start feeling better. If you are able to continue with the schedule, your persistence will be rewarded with better sleep and improved daytime functioning.

GOAL SETTING

Now that you have collected the necessary data, you can start setting some goals. In the first section of this chapter, I prompted you with questions to determine your sleep need. If, through answering those questions, you have discovered what your sleep need is, you can begin by reducing or increasing your time in bed accordingly. For instance, if you remembered that you were sleeping seven hours per night and functioning well prior to the birth of your first child, you may make it your goal to sleep seven hours per night. If you were unable to determine your sleep need, the sleep log will be helpful.

The sleep self-assessment (see page 46) helps you discover habits that may be impacting your ability to get to sleep or stay asleep. If the questions revealed anything that may be harmful for your sleep, correcting these issues might be a goal for you. If you have several things on the self-assessment that need to be corrected, begin with one or two of them that appear to be most achievable for you. It takes time to fully optimize your sleep, and sometimes our circumstances keep us from achieving all of these goals. So, just change the things that you can easily alter first, and then make plans to change the others when your life settles down.

The insomnia severity assessment (see page 113) gives you an idea of how much your insomnia is impairing normal daily functioning. If you answered any of the questions with a low score, improving that particular activity may be a goal. For instance, if you answered the question about work or volunteering with a low number because you fall asleep at your desk, you may want to make a goal to stand up and stretch or take a short walk every hour to maintain wakefulness until you're able to correct your sleep time. You may no longer have these symptoms once your sleep has been optimized.

The sleep log can be used in several ways. You may be able to detect patterns in your sleep and also calculate your average sleep. This is a good place to start with sleep-period restriction. Then, set a goal for the number of hours you spend in bed. In addition, you may notice patterns in your daytime functioning when you get a certain amount of sleep. Sometimes, that can clue you into your sleep need. You may also notice patterns in daytime functioning after you take a substance to aid sleep (sleeping pill, alcohol), which can help you set a goal about sleep aids.

If your sleep log reveals that your sleep pattern is quite variable, try setting a goal to regulate your sleep period. For example, if you notice that you're spending roughly the same time asleep every night but it takes you two hours to get to sleep, you may benefit from making it a goal to simply delay your bedtime by two hours—especially if you are functioning well during the day. Alternatively, if you're getting to sleep rapidly but waking frequently in the night, your goal may be to reduce your time in bed by the amount of time you are awake in the night. Sometimes, you can see patterns in early awakenings that help you make goals regarding your sleep period. For instance, if you go to bed at 10 p.m. and spontaneously wake up at 4 a.m. and are unable to return to sleep on many or most days per week, you may conclude that you are a six-hour sleeper.

Whatever you find, and whatever goals you set, if you continue to fill out your sleep log, you may discover new goals as you master some of your first goals. Changing your sleep habits is a process. Reward yourself when you reach a goal; it will help you maintain that habit and address other challenges in your sleep.

Finally, continue to journal. When stressors emerge in our lives, we often respond to them in similar ways. So our sleep habits can, again, be derailed when we are under stress. Knowing this prior to a stressful situation can build our awareness of potential stressors and ward them off. If you do relapse, you have a record in your journal of how you were able to normalize your sleep habits. It will help you re-optimize your sleep once again.

SELF-REFLECTION

Is there anything surprising about your baseline results? Do you feel anything is inaccurate?

_____

_____

_____

_____

_____

_____

_____

MOVING FORWARD ·

In the last three chapters, we have learned a great deal about anxiety and insomnia. We have also assessed our sleep and the habits around it. We are now ready to put this knowledge into action.

The remainder of this book is going to be spent actually practicing CBT techniques. There is often a great deal of anxiety around sleep, so we will deal with that issue first. I'll guide you through the steps of relieving your anxiety around sleep. Then we'll apply these techniques to alleviate your insomnia. I'll also lead you through the steps of correcting habits that impact sleep. It won't be easy, but it will be rewarding because you'll learn how to achieve a restful night's sleep.

PART TWO

······························

THE
PROGRAM

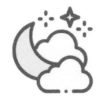

CHAPTER FOUR

Working Through Anxious Thoughts

· ·

In this chapter, we will learn how to manage and even change our thought patterns. Some of the intrusive, automatic thoughts that impair our daily lives can be corrected by changing our response to them. I will take you through a step-by-step process to help you identify those thoughts and the feelings associated with them and then provide another process for correcting them.

CHALLENGE YOUR THOUGHTS WITH CBT ·····

In order to change our thoughts, we must first identify those thoughts that cause discomfort and lower our self-confidence. Once we have identified them, we can begin the step-by-step process of challenging and altering them through reason, which may sometimes conflict with our core beliefs. This is a powerful coping skill and can help you deal with intrusive thoughts.

Identify Troubling Situations/Conditions

The first step is to identify your triggers. You might start by reviewing your current coping mechanisms (such as alcohol to self-medicate, stress eating, lashing out at others, running away from a problem/issue). If you can identify the coping mechanism, you can begin to search for triggers. What happened to cause you to reach for that beer? From what or whom do you feel like you need to run? Write down what you discover in a journal, so you have a record of your progress.

A trigger is a sudden strong emotional reaction that seems out of proportion to the situation. For instance, I was recently having a conversation on Facebook with a high school colleague who was expressing his opinion about a political matter. When I read the comment, I felt attacked because he was tearing my argument apart. I walked away from that conversation and simply did not respond. When analyzing the issue, I realized that one of my core beliefs is that the people in my hometown do not approve of my unique views on life, which is an overgeneralization. When I recognized the error in my thinking, I was able to restructure my thought patterns and gain self-confidence. I was then able to return to the conversation and respond appropriately.

Become Aware of Your Thoughts

Once you have identified a trigger, record the triggering event in your journal. Ask yourself questions about it. What happened? Who was with me when it happened? When did I first notice that I was becoming emotional about the situation? Where did it take place? Thinking of the situation in terms of the who, what, when, and where will help you find your triggers. After you have completed this exercise, read over your journal entry. Notice and record the thoughts that come up in your mind as you read about the event. Doing so will help you recognize your automatic intrusive thoughts.

Identify Negative/Inaccurate Thinking

As you analyze your thoughts, take notice of what you're feeling. How strong is your emotion? Rate your emotion on a scale of 1 to 10 (where 1 is not emotional at all and 10 is highly emotional). Document your emotion and its intensity. Sometimes, you may have more than one emotion. For instance, if you're cut off in traffic and narrowly avoid an accident, you may have a combination of anger (for being cut off) and fear (of potentially being injured in a collision).

Reshape Negative/Inaccurate Thinking

The next step is to reshape or reframe your emotion. In this step, think of alternative ways of thinking about the situation. For instance, in the traffic example, you might think to yourself, "I almost got hit, but I am a good driver, and I was able to avoid an accident. I am thankful." Document your reshaped thought. Do this for every triggered emotional experience you have recorded.

Reread and Re-rate Your Thoughts

The last step is to reread and re-rate your emotion. After you have reshaped several emotions, go back to your original emotions and read about them a second and third time. Then, re-rate them. The intensity of the emotion is likely to go down, sometimes significantly. The more you do this, the better you will get at it. In addition, as you get better with reshaping your emotions, your automatic thoughts will become more positive as well.

Downward Arrow Technique

Sometimes, it is difficult to determine where an emotion came from. Often, the underlying belief has been with us so long—operating in the back of our mind—that we have difficulty finding the trigger itself. The Downward Arrow Technique can help you discover the core belief that has triggered the emotion.

Begin by asking what your thought means. For instance, I recall thinking to myself, "No one wants to do things with me socially anymore." This caused me to feel shame, depression, and fear that seemed excessive for a problem with such a relatively simple solution. So I applied the Downward Arrow Technique to my situation. My trajectory went like this: I'm not socially active, which means that → My friends are rejecting me, which means that → I'll be sad and alone, which means that → I'm being abandoned.

This technique gets to the basic issue that is triggering your emotions. Notice the flawed thinking in this pattern. For instance, true friends do not reject you. More likely, they also have very busy lives. In discussing your loneliness with your friends, you may discover a solution. Document your findings. Write down the trajectory of your thoughts and identify the erroneous thinking. Frequent themes are about perfectionism, hopelessness, powerlessness, threat, abandonment, and injustice.

SELF-REFLECTION

Do you recall a time when anxious thoughts kept you from sleeping? What, if anything, did you do to combat these thoughts? Can you use the techniques we have discussed to reduce them? Notice if your automatic thoughts have a similar theme each night. If so, which of the techniques we've discussed so far might help you reduce these intrusive thoughts?

Managing Anxiety

CBT includes tools to help you deal with anxiety. These tools can be used in any situation, but in this book, we are concerned about anxiety and sleep. CBT techniques may not "cure" you, but they can provide you with the skills to manage anxiety in a healthy way. As you change your behavior, you'll likely become more self-confident and more positive about your ability to handle this challenge. The more you put these tools to use, the more successful you'll be at managing your anxiety and getting to sleep.

GETTING THE MOST OUT OF CBT · · · · · · · · · · · · · · · ·

There is one key element to remember as you begin to work on changing how you think: persistence. You may be trying to change many years of habitual behavior, so give yourself plenty of time and be kind to yourself as you begin practicing CBT techniques.

Approach Therapy as a Partnership

If you're choosing to apply CBT tools without the assistance of a healthcare provider, consider enlisting a good friend, family member, or partner to help you with identifying your emotions and core beliefs. You may benefit from their suggestions. If you've chosen to find a therapist, you'll get the most out of your experience if you remain an active participant in analyzing your emotions and applying CBT techniques. You may also choose to find a support group—the Anxiety and Depression Association of America lists support groups in many areas of the country.

Be Open and Honest

Make a sincere effort to be open and honest about your feelings. It's hard sometimes to maintain a close watch on your emotions, but with time and practice, you'll likely find it gets easier. When you're able to identify your emotions, you may be tempted to resist discussing certain events. As you become more adept and comfortable, you may realize that your previous resistance has melted away and you're less rigid about making changes. Be patient with yourself and continue to move forward. In the meantime, use your journal to note those things you prefer not to discuss with others, so you have a record of your insights.

Stick to the Plan

Take time to analyze your feelings and be consistent in your approach. Changing how you think takes a lot of time and effort. Don't be afraid to ask for help if you encounter something that's difficult to understand. As you work through the problem, new insights may emerge that will help you move forward. If it becomes too uncomfortable, it's okay to take a break and sit with the uneasiness. But don't quit; the more intense your effort, the more likely you will be rewarded with less anxiety and better sleep.

Don't Expect Instant Results

One of the hardest parts of CBT is continuing the program. It can be very uncomfortable to play in an unfamiliar emotional playground where you're challenging your previously "normal" behavior. Persistence is key to success—the more you practice, the easier it becomes. First, choose small, easily achievable goals. Your initial successes will give you the confidence you'll need to stick to your plan, reach your goals, and take on more challenging tasks.

Do Your Homework

Earlier, we discussed that it takes about two weeks of consistency in your sleep schedule for the brain to adjust. When we're changing deep-seated, long-held core beliefs and emotional reactions to triggers, it takes even more time. Relish the little successes you see. Record them and reward yourself for even the smallest accomplishments. Every step forward is leading you toward your goal. You won't get instant results, but if you remain persistent, you can usually reach your goals. Remember, you may be challenging lifelong beliefs and patterns, which takes time. Consider how rewarding it will be to cross the finish line.

Seek Outside Help

If you feel you've given CBT a fair chance without a therapist and are not happy with the progress you're making, consider getting the help of a therapist in your area. Find a person you feel you can work well with and with whom you'll feel comfortable discussing your emotions. Therapists often assign activities outside the therapy session that can help address the issues you're working on together. They also may have further resources for you to explore, some of which may include variations of the other therapies we will discuss in the next section.

OTHER THERAPIES FOR ANXIETY ················

One of the most common ways of dealing with anxiety is to take medication for it. As we discussed in chapter 2 (see page 32), medications for sleep often work for a short period of time until the body becomes accustomed to them, and then changes in medication need to be made. In addition, many medications for anxiety are habit forming and can be very difficult to stop. While medication is sometimes necessary, in most cases, CBT is a better option.

There are over-the-counter supplements that can help with anxiety. Unfortunately, many of these supplements interfere with medications used for other illnesses. For example, St. John's wort may be very effective in dealing with anxiety issues, but if you are on any prescription medication, it is likely to interact with that medication, making it either less effective or enhancing the effects of the drug. Both can be dangerous.

For some people, aromatherapy is helpful for calming the anxious mind. Lavender oil can help you relax and get to sleep. RutaVaLa contains valerian and lavender, and it can be very calming when used in a diffuser. Chamomile has a similar effect when the oil is diffused or made into tea during stressful periods. Finally, vetiver can be diffused for a soothing effect and also has a lovely aroma.

There are a few other therapies that are designed to calm anxiety, reduce stress, and achieve emotional balance. I will discuss each below. If you decide to pursue one of these therapies, choose one that seems most natural to you. Attempting to do something that doesn't seem natural may increase your stress.

Exercise

Exercise has long been known to relieve anxiety. It is thought to help support and enhance the coping mechanisms used during stressful times. Studies show that individuals who exercise regularly find a significant amount of relief from their symptoms. A 2010 study in *Psychology of Sport and Exercise* found that exercise in natural spaces enhances this resolution of symptoms. A 2013 study in the *British Journal of Sports Medicine* found that both aerobic and anaerobic exercise were effective in relieving stress and anxiety.

Relaxation Techniques

Following thought-challenging exercises with a relaxation technique may slow your mind and allow it to reset. Mindfulness is helpful when you're able to focus on something other than the thoughts that are passing through your mind. Meditation, similarly, keeps your mind occupied with your breath. Visual imagery can also be effective, especially when used in conjunction with meditation. Progressive muscle relaxation puts the muscles in a more relaxed state, which aids in relaxing your mind.

Biofeedback

Biofeedback uses instruments to measure your body's response to stress. A therapist analyzes the results, giving you a better understanding of what your body is doing and what to look for when you're going through a stressful situation. For instance, it can tell you if your heart rate increases, if your muscles tense, if you begin to sweat or have clammy hands, if your breathing rate increases, etc. Biofeedback can help you discover these clues and regulate your response to stress.

Hypnosis

The goal of hypnosis is to remove the association of environmental triggers from the anxiety response. During hypnosis, the mind is more relaxed and better able to respond to suggestions. Hypnosis can be used to uncover past traumatic events, which then helps you understand the origin of your anxiety triggers. This gives you clues about the automatic thoughts and core beliefs that you can work on using the tools you have learned.

COMPLEMENTARY ALTERNATIVE MEDICINES

Have you tried any other therapies or methods to combat anxiety? Which ones, and what were the results?

_____

_____

_____

_____

_____

MOVING FORWARD

Now that we've seen how CBT works in the treatment of anxiety, in the next chapter we'll explore how CBT-I techniques work to improve insomnia. We'll discuss multiple behavioral elements that can optimize your ability to get to sleep and stay asleep as you apply CBT-I methods.

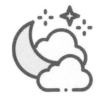

CHAPTER FIVE

CBT-I: There is Help for Insomnia

· · · · · · · · · · · ·

In this chapter, we will discuss applying CBT-I techniques to manage insomnia. Many of the behaviors that we have developed over the course of a lifetime can impair our ability to get to sleep and stay asleep. Taking on the challenge of insomnia is a process. It took you many years of detrimental habits and behaviors to get you here today, so it will probably also take some time to turn it around. We turn, now, to the techniques of CBT-I to help with this process.

TURNING TO CBT-I ·······································

Our behaviors around sleep have the potential of helping us get to sleep and stay asleep at night. These behaviors will also involve our daytime activities. When we make sleep a priority, we learn to balance those things that can reduce our ability to get to sleep and stay asleep with those activities that can promote good sleep. CBT-I works with the following factors. Later in this chapter we will go into further detail for each.

Sleep Hygiene: Sleep hygiene refers to a group of behaviors that can enhance your sleep experience. The most important aspect of sleep hygiene is regulation of the sleep period. This means going to bed at the same time every night and getting up at the same time every morning. Other important sleep hygiene factors include the timing of your exercise routine and the last and first meals of the day, the use of caffeine and tobacco, and your bedtime routine.

Sleep Restriction: Sleep restriction is simply spending only enough time in bed to fulfill your sleep need. In chapter 3, you learned how much time you need to spend in bed. Putting this sleep schedule into place and only spending enough time in bed to get adequate sleep is important. When you look at your bed, it's important that your mind is thinking about sleep (intimacy and sickness are the only exceptions).

Stimulus Control: Another important component of CBT-I is stimulus control, which means managing your sleep environment so that outside stimuli don't interfere with sleep. I like to think of this part as an invitation to sleep. You're making everything in your environment conducive to sleep as though you're inviting sleep as a guest in your bedroom. Inviting sleep involves several things:

- Making your bedroom environment cool, quiet, dark, and comfortable

- Reducing screen time prior to bedtime

- Optimizing the timing of exercise and your evening meal

Sleep-Interfering Arousal/Activation: Sleep arousal refers to the daily stressors and worries that we often take to bed with us at night. Reducing sleep-interfering activation involves calming the mind—using the techniques I have previously mentioned (see page 35)—and changing our thought patterns to recognize that we cannot force sleep. We must allow sleep to come to us.

Food and Substances: Substances that we put into our bodies can interfere with our ability to stay asleep or quickly reach deeper stages of sleep. This is important because if you're able to get into the deeper stages of sleep quickly, you'll also be able to stay asleep much more easily. These substances, which we will elaborate on later (see page 90), stimulate the brain.

Foods can also have a significant effect on sleep. Our body's core temperature needs to be cooler to get to sleep easily. Eating within four hours of bedtime can increase the blood supply to our core in order to digest food, which warms the body and reduces our ability to get to sleep quickly. We will discuss how to plan meals around bedtime and wake time later in this chapter (see page 91).

Biological Clock: We are each born with a biological clock that determines the timing of our sleep period. Our biological clock actually has two sleep phases: our nighttime phase, and a sleep dip that occurs anytime between 11 a.m. and 3 p.m., depending on your sleep timing. This is a natural time of day to sleep, which is why the world's siesta societies nap at this time. It also makes the timing of meals an important component of sleep hygiene. There are moments when eating a small snack before bedtime is appropriate, but this is generally not the case.

IDENTIFYING NEGATIVE THOUGHT PATTERNS

Think about your feelings as you prepare for sleep. Can you identify some behaviors that reinforce negative thinking about sleep? Using the techniques discussed in chapter 4, write down your behaviors, identify the emotion, and rate the strength of this emotion. Over the next few days, read over these emotions and re-rate their strength. Gradually, these emotions will get weaker, and you may find that sleep comes more easily.

_____

_____

_____

_____

_____

_____

_____

_____

_____

_____

_____

_____

_____

SLEEP HYGIENE ·························

Sleep hygiene consists of a group of behaviors, environmental conditions, and other factors—many of which are well-known—that can affect your ability to sleep at the appropriate time. Adjusting our behaviors to invite sleep can help remove the environmental barriers to achieving it.

Look at your sleep self-assessment. Which sleep habits need optimization? We will further discuss many of these issues here.

Sleep Schedule

When we send parents home from the hospital with a new baby, one of the first things we tell them to do is to put the child on a schedule. Doing the same things at roughly the same time every day will help the child acclimate to daily rituals. When we become adults, we often choose to avoid following a daily schedule, and when we are young and resilient, this may have few negative effects. But with age, we become less resilient and are more likely to require a schedule.

The most important part of your sleep schedule is the wake time, which is the time that your biological day begins. Keeping it stable will make it considerably easier to achieve sleep. You determined what your sleep need is in chapter 3 (see page 43). To set your sleep schedule, simply determine your earliest wake time during the week and set that as your daily wake time. Working backward will help you set your bedtime. If you need to be up at 5 a.m. every day and your sleep need is seven hours, you would want to go to bed at 10 p.m. Because we generally don't sleep the entire time we're in bed, I recommend adding 30 to 60 minutes to your sleep need. In the example above, the bedtime should be between 9 p.m. and 9:30 p.m.

If you're not sleepy at your bedtime, wait until you feel sleepy before you go to bed. This means you may occasionally have a short night because you still need to get out of bed at your wake time. But that's actually a good thing because your sleep drive should be very strong the next night, and you should be able to get to sleep more easily. Avoid catastrophizing when you have a short night—you've had them many times before, and you survived. Just a few more of them, and sleep will be answering your invitation.

Don't Linger

If you're lying in bed and you're getting uncomfortable, get out of bed. Take your racing thoughts to another room and do something dull, boring, and monotonous under dim light until you get sleepy. When you feel sleepy, go back to bed and try again. This will move your rumination from the bedroom to a more appropriate place. Similarly, in the morning, don't lie in bed for more than a few minutes, and especially not long enough to begin thinking about your day.

If you're prone to watching the clock, turn it away from you. The only thing you need from your clock is the alarm. Seeing numbers often gets us thinking or doing nighttime math. When we do that, our emotions often get involved, making it even more difficult to return to sleep. Avoiding this problem by turning the clock away is a better solution.

Engage Your Space

Think about your mattress, pillows, and what you wear to bed. Are they comfortable for you? Discomfort can invite negative thoughts and perceptions of sleep. Is your bedroom cool? Quiet? Dark? These are conditions that typically invite sleep and reduce sleep disturbances.

Napping

As a general rule, avoid napping during the day. Napping often reduces your sleep drive at night, when it's most needed. If you absolutely feel like you need a nap, take it before 3 p.m. for 30 minutes or less. Typically, that amount of rest will not interfere with your nighttime sleep drive.

Entertain Outside the Bedroom

Another rule of thumb is to keep your bed for only sleep, intimacy, and sickness. Anything else tells the brain that it is acceptable to do things other than sleep in bed. Reading in bed (even without a screen) is generally not a good idea. Instead, read in a comfortable chair beside the bed until you get sleepy, and then simply crawl into your bed and turn out the lights. In addition, avoid screens (TV, cell phone, tablet, computer) one hour prior to bedtime.

Monitor Substances

Nicotine and caffeine are stimulants. Similar to light, they keep the brain from reaching the deeper stages of sleep quickly. Caffeine stays in our systems for 10 to 12 hours, so I recommend no caffeine within eight hours of bedtime. Nicotine is shorter acting, so avoiding it four hours prior to bedtime is a good rule of thumb. Alcohol is a depressant and can make you sleepy because it enters the bloodstream very rapidly. But it also leaves the bloodstream quickly and can wake you up about four hours after ingestion. You may not wake to full consciousness, but you may also feel sleepier than normal the following morning after having alcohol close to bedtime because it has limited your deep sleep. Getting into the deep stages of sleep quickly helps keep us asleep, and there are also many significant health benefits in the deeper stages of sleep as we learned in chapter 1 (see page 3).

Reducing Screen Time

The reason screens cause problems with sleep is because they stimulate the brain. The photoreceptors in our eyes react when they encounter light, and the ray that these photoreceptors respond to most strongly is the blue ray. Our brain is then stimulated to wake up because blue light interferes with melatonin production. As you may recall, melatonin is one of the hormones that our biological clock uses to help us get to sleep. Therefore, reducing screen time prior to bedtime will increase melatonin production and enhance sleep. Many people can get to sleep after using screens, but they are typically unable to achieve deep sleep quickly. A 2013 study in the *Journal of Sleep Research* shows that evening exposure to light delays our ability to get into non-REM sleep in the early part of the night. In other words, it delays the onset of the deeper stages of sleep.

TRY IT

The most important aspect of sleep hygiene is regulation of the sleep schedule. For two weeks, try getting out of bed at the same time every day. Yes, even on your days off. And yes, even if you went to bed too late. Write down how it went. What were your barriers? What challenges did you face? Were you empowered by doing something to improve your sleep? It's okay if you weren't successful. It took you a long time to get to where you are now, and it will take some time to get into a healthy sleep pattern. Give yourself a pat on the back for your efforts!

BEST LAID PLANS ·····························

Sometimes, life gets in the way, and we're unable to maintain a routine. A sleep log is one of the best ways to recognize that you are resuming previous behaviors. If you periodically review your sleep patterns, you may be able to adjust early to any changes that may be taking place in your sleep as a result of life stressors.

At other times, we get so caught up in our stressors and what we need to do to meet the current situation that we quickly revert back to our old patterns of behavior. This is normal. As soon as you realize what's happening, go back to your journal and see how you handled similar situations in the past. And remember, you're changing the associations your brain makes through CBT-I. This takes time, so give yourself credit for recognizing where you are and for restarting your program.

If you haven't recorded your progress or you find yourself in a new situation that you haven't yet experienced, plan your strategy and be sure to write it down. Make use of the CBT tools you learned in chapter 4 (see page 61) if anxiety is ramping up. By now, you have likely learned to keep your mind open to any possibility, regardless of how farfetched it seems. Sometimes, reviewing your journal and seeing the progress you have already made will give you the self-confidence to continue despite any setbacks.

When work schedules get in the way of bedtime, or if you have small children that frequently awaken in the night, you may be tempted to spend more time in bed. Don't give in to the temptation. This may mean you'll have a sleepy day, but, as I've said, you have done this before, and you can get through it again. Remember, one sleepy day is a whole lot easier to manage than a week's or month's worth of sleepy days. Continue to get up at your regular wake time and console yourself with the thought that your next night of sleep will be awesome because your sleep drive will be high.

STRATEGIES FOR STAYING ASLEEP

Sometimes, even if you have restricted your sleep, you may find it difficult to stay asleep or get back to sleep. In general, restricting your time in bed typically manages this aspect of sleep, but if you have other medical issues (pain, urinary tract infection, prostate issues), sleep can often be interrupted. Environmental factors (pets, children, bed partner) may also interfere with sleep, but avoid allowing your emotions to emerge during these times. The longer you let anxiety or anger fester, the harder it will be to get back to sleep.

Progressive relaxation or deep breathing can often help in these situations. Meditation is also a great tool. Often, you are lying down so that relaxation, along with counting of your breaths, can lead you back into slumber.

Avoid anything active at this time. The more active you are, the higher the chance will be that you'll wake up more and have difficulty returning to sleep. Avoid turning on lights as well. It will be easier to get back to sleep if you use night lights to navigate when you are up in the night. Avoid looking at the clock; that often gets your mind moving as well. Try using the ritual that you use to get to sleep or some other tool that works better in the night. Remain quiet, calm, and invite sleep in once again.

If you're unable to get to sleep and you're getting uncomfortable resting in your bed, get out of bed. Go to another room and do something you know will make you sleepy, and then try again. Get up at your normal wake time.

If sleeplessness is becoming a pattern, record the presumed amount of time you were awake and shorten your sleep period by that amount of time. The results of our sleep-need analysis are not always exact and sometimes need adjustment. But only change your sleep time by 15 minutes at a time. For instance, if you wake in the night and are consistently awake for 30 minutes, reduce your time in bed by 15 minutes for two weeks. If you feel better, you're all set. If not, try reducing it again by another 15 minutes.

SELF-REFLECTION

Have you tried any of the sleep hygiene techniques to improve your sleep? If so, was it easy for you, or did you run into barriers? Were you able to manage the challenges? If so, how?

_____

_____

_____

_____

_____

_____

SLEEP RESTRICTION & EFFICIENCY ·············

Remember, sleep restriction refers to the amount of time you spend in bed in relation to the amount of time you're actually sleeping.

Practicing Restriction

Sleep restriction can be a time-consuming process, but in time, you will determine your ideal sleep need. Once you find your schedule, you will likely gradually feel better over the course of a year. At that point, you may also feel more stable and know better how to manage any issues that threaten the stability of your sleep schedule. In addition, you will develop coping mechanisms for your most challenging tasks. Continue to journal as you make changes so that you can go back to your notes should you ever need to.

At first, when you restrict your time in bed, you may be spending more time awake in or outside of your bed than normal. This works in your favor because the more time you spend awake on any given night, the stronger your sleep drive will be the next night. The more effort you put into adjusting your sleep schedule, the quicker this will happen for you.

Gaining Efficiency

As you reduce your time in bed and increase the number of hours in bed that you are sleeping, you are also increasing your sleep efficiency. Sleep efficiency is calculated by taking the actual sleep time and dividing it by the number of hours you spend in bed. A normal sleep efficiency is regarded as 85 percent or higher.

HOW TO INCREASE/REDUCE YOUR TIME IN BED

If you continue to have some insomnia symptoms, reduce your time in bed by 15 minutes every two weeks until the insomnia issues resolve. At that point, stay at your current schedule. Don't be afraid to make changes to see if you can improve your sleep efficiency and reduce your insomnia symptoms. Remember that it takes time to set a new schedule in motion.

If you are still feeling sleepy after about one month of practicing sleep period restriction, you can change your sleep schedule as needed. If you feel like you need more time in bed, every two weeks add 15 minutes per day to your sleep period, and see how you feel. When you begin to have difficulty getting to sleep or staying asleep over a significant period of time (typically two weeks), you may, once again, be spending too much time in bed. At this point, revert to your prior schedule. For instance, if you have increased your time in bed from 6.5 hours to 6.75 hours and you begin to have difficulty getting to sleep or staying asleep, go back to your 6.5-hour schedule.

STIMULUS CONTROL

Stimulus control is about adjusting your sleep environment and sleep practices to promote relaxation and avoid excess activity, which helps invite sleep. Preparing your body and brain for sleep can have a profound effect on your ability to get to sleep and stay asleep. Your brain may currently be trained so that you can do many activities in bed because that has been your experience in the past. You now need to retrain your brain. We do this by controlling our behaviors around sleep and in the bedroom and by developing a set of repetitive activities prior to sleep so that the brain can make new associations. There are several techniques that can help you usher in sleep. The more you practice these techniques, the more your brain will associate them with preparation for sleep.

Get Out of Bed

The first technique is to train yourself to think "sleep" when you look at your bed. If you do anything in bed other than sleep, intimacy, or rest due to sickness, your mind has been conditioned to associate those activities rather than sleep with bed. To strengthen your brain's association between your bed and "sleep," you'll need to avoid doing anything in bed other than sleep. Even reading in bed is risky—this is especially true if you habitually fall asleep reading with the lights on; the light stimulation changes the architecture of your sleep. I suggest that you place a chair beside your bed or somewhere in your bedroom and read there under dim light until you get sleepy.

Develop a Routine

Develop a nighttime routine in which you have completed all busy activities (brushing teeth, brushing hair, showering, putting pajamas on, and turning the bed down) about one hour before bedtime. After you have done your active tasks, do something for 30 to 45 minutes that you find very calming and relaxing. Avoid screens during this time, and if you read, avoid the material that you have difficulty putting down. Instead, choose something that you can set aside at any time but that is interesting enough to you to keep you awake until your scheduled bedtime. Doing this every night will be a signal to your brain, over time, that you are preparing for sleep.

Go to Bed When Sleepy

Only go to bed when you are feeling sleepy. If you aren't sleepy at your bedtime, wait until you get sleepy, and go to bed at that time. Generally, if we are not sleepy when we go to bed, we often bring with us all of the thoughts, ruminations, and concerns about our previous day or the following day. This is not acceptable in bed, and if you catch yourself doing it, simply get out of bed and take these issues to another room. Keep the lights low and don't do anything stimulating—dull and boring are your friends now. This process should also be used if you wake up in the night and find yourself thinking about past or future events. You are training your brain to determine what is acceptable in bed.

Morning Rise Time

Choose a wake time and get up at that time every day of the week. Your circadian sleep drive begins when you wake up in the morning. Maintaining a stable start every day will help you get to sleep better at your scheduled bedtime. The more stability you have in your sleep schedule, the easier it will be to go to sleep and stay asleep.

BREATHING IN BED

A good practice when trying to relax in bed is diaphragmatic breathing. With this technique, you take slow, deep breaths from the diaphragm. Your stomach should move up with each inhalation and down with each exhalation. Slowing your breathing will signal your mind to also slow down. When you have taken a few relaxing breaths, imagine a place where you feel relaxed. It may be the beach or a forest. What do you smell? What do you see? Is it warm? Do you feel the sun warming your skin? Do you hear ocean waves? Or squirrels rustling in the leaves?

SLEEP-INTERFERING AROUSAL/ACTIVATION

There are some daily activities that can interfere with sleep. Adjusting our schedules so that these activities don't happen too close to bedtime can help the body relax enough to get to sleep. In addition, there are other activities that reduce sensory input and, therefore, may help invite sleep.

Unwind Before Bed

If you're under a great deal of stress or are having anxiety issues prior to bedtime, try some of the CBT techniques discussed in chapter 4 (see page 61). Mindfulness can be especially helpful because it turns your focus onto your body and the external cues around you rather than allowing your mind to bring up intrusive thoughts. Relaxation and breathing techniques can also be beneficial.

Proper Sleep Environment

Adjusting the cues in your environment can also usher in sleep. If you're sensitive to smell, you might try diffusing some calming oils or getting some lotions that have a calming scent. If you have sensitive hearing, you may want to have some white or pink noise in your bedroom to reduce auditory input. While both white and pink noise are easily heard by the human ear, pink noise is smoother because its intensity decreases as the frequency of the noise increases. White noise can be something as simple as running a fan in your bedroom. There are white noise machines, apps, and CDs that can be purchased. Pink noise, a relatively new phenomenon, can also be found online and in smartphone apps. Choose a sound that is calming and relaxing for you.

Problem-Solve

If you consistently have a particular topic come up as you're trying to sleep, you may wish to preempt it by simply doing something about it. For example, if you are worrying about having the children's lunches ready in time for them to leave for school, plan to put the lunches together before bedtime. You have solved the problem and saved a little time for your next day. This allows your brain to invite sleep.

Avoid Exercise Too Close to Bedtime

Regular exercise is good for the body and will also help you sleep, but the timing of exercise is very important. For those who have difficulty getting to sleep, exercise works best first thing in the morning. It gets your body moving and helps wake you up. If you continue to be active after your morning exercise, your body and mind will remain stimulated during the day as long as you continue your activities. If exercise does not fit into your morning schedule, be sure to complete your exercise routine at least four hours before bedtime. This will allow enough time for your body to relax and for your body's core to cool.

The Pavlov Connection

Pavlovian theory describes how the stimuli in our environment helps us make associations in our brain. Pavlov's dogs learned to associate the sight of food and the sound of a bell to being fed, and they would begin to salivate. The principle is similar with sleep. The more stimuli we can train our brain to associate with planning to sleep, the easier it will be to get to sleep. This is also why the bed should only be for sleep (and intimacy and sickness). If you only sleep in bed, your brain will begin to think "sleep" when you lie down, making it easier for sleep to come to you.

The exercises discussed earlier—building a nighttime routine, taking any ruminations or thoughts out of your bedroom, getting out of bed if you cannot get to sleep, avoiding screens—are all designed to provide additional associations for your brain. If you are able to do these things consistently, your brain will begin to relax, and your nighttime relaxing routine will begin to make you sleepy. If you regularly use a fan or diffuse oils at your bedside, your brain will also associate those with sleep, making the process much easier.

STRESS-REDUCTION ACTIVITIES

Think about any sleep-interfering activities you may be doing before bed-time that could be unhelpful. Now, think of three to four helpful activities that you could do to unwind from stress. Will these activities alert your brain that you're preparing for sleep? Try to choose activities that you can perform only when you're preparing for sleep.

WHAT YOU PUT IN YOUR BODY ···················

Substances that you put in your body throughout the course of an entire day can affect your sleep. In addition, when you consume these substances is important. To optimize your sleep, you will want to pay attention to what time you consume alcohol, stimulating substances, and food.

Alcohol

Many people self-medicate with alcohol to get to sleep at night. Alcohol is a depressant, so it often helps. But alcohol enters and leaves the bloodstream rapidly, which means that about four hours after you stop drinking alcohol, it will quickly leave your system with the opposite effect. It can wake you up or, at least, bump you out of the deeper, more restorative stages of sleep. Either way, alcohol fragments your sleep, so you won't feel as rested when you wake up in the morning.

Stimulants

Caffeine stays in your system for 10 to 12 hours. It's a stimulant and can keep you awake. I generally recommend no caffeine eight hours before bedtime because it lingers in the body. You may be able to get to sleep after having caffeine, but you will likely have difficulty getting into the deeper stages of sleep rapidly, and the changes in your sleep architecture can make you feel more tired the next day.

Many people only associate caffeine with coffee, but many other foods, beverages, and over-the-counter medications contain caffeine as well. Though the name suggests otherwise, even decaffeinated coffee contains caffeine, albeit much less than regular coffee. Tea contains roughly half the amount of caffeine as coffee. Chocolate and hot cocoa contain caffeine because there is a significant amount of caffeine in cacao beans (from which chocolate is made). But it's not always as stimulating as some of the other sources of caffeine because of its chemical composition. Even breakfast cereals, pudding, frozen yogurt, and ice cream contain caffeine—especially the chocolate-flavored varieties.

Medications used for premenstrual syndrome (PMS) often contain caffeine, as do some headache pain relievers.

Surprising to some, nicotine is, in fact, a stimulant. It does not stay in the system as long as caffeine does, but people should avoid tobacco four hours before bedtime because it stimulates the brain.

Eating at Night

If you eat a heavy meal in the evening, the timing of your meal is important. Digestion uses energy and warms the body's core, especially when you eat proteins. That means you'll want to eat your meal about four hours before bedtime to allow plenty of time for digestion and for the body to cool in preparation for sleep. You could also opt for a lighter meal in the evening—something that is easy to digest but filling enough to keep you asleep. For those who wake up in the night feeling hungry, a small snack before bedtime may be necessary to stave off hunger until morning. If you snack prior to bedtime, be sure it is something light like a piece of fruit.

Eating high-carbohydrate meals often cause sleepiness, typically because of their sugar content. Sugar can give you a burst of energy, but it is also short-lived, and a fast reduction in sugars can cause significant sleepiness. Choosing a low-carbohydrate meal, especially at lunch time, will help you more easily stay awake. When we have a high-carbohydrate lunch before or during our sleep dip, we are more likely to get intensely sleepy.

BIOLOGICAL CLOCK

The biological clock determines the time of day that it is most natural for you to sleep. Some consider themselves morning people (larks); they wake up, jump out of bed, and are ready to start their day. Others are night people (owls); they have difficulty waking in the morning but can often easily stay up till the wee hours of the morning. Still others are neither owls nor larks; they wake up not as energetic as morning people but with enough energy to get their day started easily. They don't like to go to bed early but would also find it difficult to stay up too late.

The biological clock works with sleep homeostasis (balance in our wake/sleep rhythm) to regulate sleep. When we compare a short sleeper who is a night owl with a normal sleeper, they may get up at the same time every morning, but the night owl went to bed much later than the normal sleeper. Sometimes, there is a mismatch between our biological clock and what is required in our daily lives. The night owl who is a normal sleeper timewise but who also needs to be at work at 7 a.m. is a good example. His natural biological clock compels him to stay up until 1 a.m., but he is an eight-hour sleeper. So, he loses out on several hours of sleep if he maintains his natural sleep habits because he needs to get out of bed early and, therefore, cannot spend enough time in bed to satisfy his sleep need.

It can be very difficult to change your biological clock, but there are ways. The two main regulators of sleep in the body are melatonin and light. The easiest and quickest way for the night owl in the above example to adjust his circadian clock would be simply to stay up all night one night and go to bed the following night at the desired bedtime. This is often unrealistic in today's society because social obligations don't allow us to take advantage of that simple remedy of staying up for an entire night.

A gradual schedule shift is likely a better option for most night owls who need to get to sleep more quickly and rise from sleep earlier than their biological clock prefers. The night owl could begin going to bed one hour earlier every three to seven days until he gets to his desired bedtime. That means he would begin by going to bed at midnight for three to seven days, then 11 p.m. for three to seven days, etc. This allows the body to adjust gradually to the change in timing of bedtime.

Another way to adjust the biological clock is by using melatonin. Individuals who are not night owls or larks typically begin secreting melatonin from the pineal gland in the brain at around 7 p.m. Taking immediate-release melatonin at that time can gradually change the circadian clock by mimicking the timing of melatonin in people who are night owls. The ideal time for our night owl in the above example to go to bed would likely be around 9:30 to 10 p.m. As a night owl, he has difficulty spontaneously getting to sleep at that hour. Employing all of our sleep hygiene and stimulus control techniques, we then add melatonin and light, which, if scheduled correctly, can adjust the body's clock.

The second thing our night owl should do is obtain exposure to light immediately after waking up in the morning. Sunlight is ideal, but turning on all lights in the rooms you're in can work too. There are also commercial light boxes that can be used for this purpose. These light boxes are similar to those currently used for seasonal affective disorder. You can find them online by searching for "light box therapy."

Finally, the night owl should maintain good sleep hygiene and continue using the techniques to control external stimuli until he takes a job more in line with his circadian rhythm. It is especially important for someone who is changing their biological clock to maintain their sleep schedule. Again, it can take weeks or months for these changes to finally feel comfortable, but gradually it can happen.

PUTTING THE PIECES TOGETHER ················

Now that you know all the steps to CBT and CBT-I techniques, you can use them to reduce your anxiety around sleep and increase your natural inclination to go to sleep. You now know what issues impair your sleep, reduce your ability to fall asleep, and interfere with your body's ability to maintain sleep. You have seen the tools that are used to deal with each of these issues, so you just need to match the problem with the appropriate tool to get started.

Whatever trouble you face or tools you choose to rectify the issue, repetition is key to resolving or reducing the problem. The more you use each of these tools, the easier it will become and the more successful you will be. Again, persistence is pivotal with CBT and CBT-I techniques.

Begin with the problems that you feel are least challenging and with which you think you'll have the most success. This way, you'll have some successes and experience prior to tackling the more difficult issues. There is only one exception to this rule: regulation of the sleep period. This should always be one of the first things to manage because it'll have a profound effect on your ability to get to sleep and stay asleep.

Don't Fight It

If you're prone to anxiety, intrusive thoughts are bound to come up. Don't fret about it; instead, take note of it and begin using the CBT tools to alter your thinking. If you tend to get anxious in the evening before bedtime because you feel "performance anxiety," mindfulness exercises can help. You can also meditate and use visual imagery to release anxious thoughts. Try to avoid catastrophizing because once your emotions get involved, it becomes harder to release the thought and get to sleep. There are many apps geared toward sleep or meditation that can help.

Designated Worry Time

We don't stop worrying just because we now have the tools to reduce it. Life brings us challenges, and some of those are worrisome. A technique to manage worry is to set aside two 15-minute periods every day just for worry. Avoid thinking about positive solutions or alternatives; just focus solely on those things that are worrying you. At the end of your worry time, take several deep, cleansing breaths as you let your worries disappear.

Don't Force Sleep

We cannot force sleep, unless we do so with substances. Your body will sleep when it needs sleep, which can cause you to fall asleep at inopportune times. This is why it is important to be proactive about it. Attempting to force sleep usually ends in frustration, anxiety, and depressive thoughts, and we often become dependent on the solution we are using (typically medications, supplements, or alcohol). Relaxation techniques, especially while lying in bed, are sometimes helpful in allowing sleep to come. A nighttime routine, if you have not yet established one, can be highly successful in helping you get to sleep.

Be in the Moment

I have mentioned mindfulness quite frequently. The technique of staying in the moment and paying attention only to our environment, not our thoughts, enhances our daily experience and helps usher in relaxation, happiness, and, ultimately, sleep. In this sense, we can also pay attention to our biologic rhythms, and if we notice anything amiss, we can take steps to address the issue. For instance, if you catch yourself thinking about the past or future, or if you're suddenly breathing rapidly, being mindful of your reaction can remind you to slow your breathing, which will often slow your mind as well. The body scan exercise is very helpful in teaching your brain to be mindful.

BODY SCAN

The body scan is a tool to help you become more attuned to and mindful of your body and its sensations. Find a comfortable place to lie down and close your eyes unless you feel you might fall asleep. Begin diaphragmatic breathing (breathing from the diaphragm) and take slow, deep breaths. Then, focus on your right toe, breathing into it. Notice any sensations in your right toe; if your mind wanders, bring your attention back to your right toe. Then, move your focus to the sole of your right foot. Feel the sensations there, the pressure of your socks on your sole. Continue this exercise over every region of your body—left leg, trunk, arms, and head. If practiced regularly, this exercise can help with the technique of mindfulness.

YOUR INDIVIDUALIZED SLEEP PLAN ·············

You've learned a lot about sleep, the multiple habits and behaviors that affect our ability to get to sleep and stay asleep, and how to manage sleep. It's now time to put all that knowledge to use and make a sleep plan. By now, you have likely determined what your sleep need is (see page 44). If so, add 30 to 60 minutes to it, and that will be the amount of time you spend in bed.

Next, you'll need to determine your wake time. What is the earliest time you have to get out of bed on any given day during the week? When you have decided your wake time, work backward from your wake time the number of hours you spend in bed. For instance, if you are a six-hour sleeper and you need to get up at 5 a.m., you'll want to spend no more than seven hours in bed. Working backwards from 5 a.m., your bedtime will be set for 10 p.m. to 10:30 p.m.

Now that you've created your sleep schedule, set an alarm for your scheduled wake time. Do not use the snooze button because it fragments your sleep and tells your brain that you don't have to follow schedules. If you have difficulty getting up despite use of your alarm, place it on the other side of the room so that you'll need to get out of bed to silence it. Then, don't go back to bed. Spend no more than 15 minutes in bed after your alarm goes off. You could consider using smart alarms if you tend to set multiple alarms. These alarms monitor your sleep cycles and wake you at the best time so that you can feel refreshed. You can read about them online by searching "smart alarms."

Now, you can set the time for your pre-sleep routine. In the example above, 9 p.m. would be a good time to get all of your active preparations for bed started. Screen time should also end at this time. By 9:15 p.m. or 9:30 p.m., you should be able to do that calming activity that helps you relax prior to sleep.

Next, pay attention to your daily behaviors that can impair sleep. Set a time for the last intake of caffeine (eight hours before bedtime), tobacco (four hours before bedtime), and when you need to have exercise completed (four hours before bedtime).

Eat your evening meal four hours prior to bedtime, particularly if it's a heavy or large meal. In the above example, you should be done eating at 6 p.m. Breakfast is the body's cue to wake up in the morning, so having a regular breakfast is also important. It should be consumed within one to two hours of waking up.

Now, you are ready to begin your journey toward healthy sleep. Remember the tools that you have learned as you embark on this journey. They are available if you need them. Track in your journal how often you use them. You may be pleasantly surprised at how much the need decreases over time.

MY SLEEP PLAN

Below is your sample sleep plan. Fill in the blank spaces with your initial sleep plan, using the parenthetical examples as a guide.

My sleep need: _____ (hours)

My time in bed: _____ (6.5 to 7 hours)

My wake time: _____ (5 a.m.)

My bedtime: _____ (10 p.m. to 10:30 p.m.)

My pre-sleep routine begins and my screen time ends at: _____ (9 p.m.)

My caffeine intake ends at: _____ (2 p.m.)

My tobacco intake ends at: _____ (6 p.m.)

My exercise routine stops at: _____ (6 p.m.)

My evening meal is completed at: _____ (6 p.m.)

My breakfast meal is started before: _____ (7 a.m.)

ASSESSMENT REVISITED ·

In your sleep plan, you've determined an appropriate bedtime and wake time. Is it significantly different than the time you were spending in bed prior to going through this workbook? As you begin to spend the appropriate time in bed, monitor the amount of time you are awake in bed without using the clock.

You can use the following questions to assess your progress:

- Did you wake in the night? How long were you awake? Is that time decreasing as you continue to follow your sleep plan?

- What barriers did you find in managing sleep hygiene? Was it difficult to stop screen time?

- Did you catch your mind racing at bedtime? If so, did you use some of the CBT tools to calm your mind?

- Did you nap during the day? If so, was it harder to get to sleep on the nights after you napped? Or did you have a short nap prior to 3 p.m.? Did you feel better or worse after your nap?

- Did pain interfere with your sleep? Did pets or children wake you up in the night? Did you find it hard to return to sleep?

- Did you find it difficult to get up at your scheduled wake time? If so, did anything help you achieve success? Can you repeat that if you were successful? Did you need to cancel any daytime activities because you were too tired to do them?

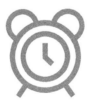

SELF-REFLECTION

Review your journal and note the progress you've made so far. Where were you successful? Give yourself a pat on the back for every success you've had, regardless of how minor it seems. Relearning sleep habits is a process, and you've made the first steps down that road. Write down your successes and celebrate them.

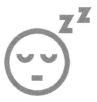

_____

_____

_____

_____

_____

_____

_____

_____

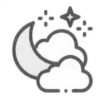

CHAPTER SIX

Committing to Change

· ·

Managing anxiety by itself is a challenge. Dealing with insomnia is equally challenging. If you're trying to address both of these issues at once, it can feel overwhelming. Challenging negative thoughts is not only important in dealing with anxiety, but can also be important in many areas of your life. You may find that as you employ the tools in this book, other problematic areas in your life begin to resolve. You may also find that as you feel more refreshed when you wake up in the morning, you have more energy to continue to use the coping skills you've learned here. My hope is that the tools that you've learned in this book will help you develop permanent coping mechanisms to meet and surpass the challenges of insomnia and anxiety.

TROUBLESHOOTING $\cdots\cdots\cdots\cdots\cdots\cdots\cdots\cdots\cdots\cdots\cdots\cdots\cdots\cdots$

When you hit a barrier to progress, try to determine if it is an anxiety-based issue or a sleep problem. Use CBT techniques to address anxiety and CBT-I techniques to manage insomnia. These can sometimes be difficult to distinguish. You also may simply try one or the other if you're unsure. If it works, problem solved. If not, move on to the other option.

One of the most common roadblocks to managing anxiety and insomnia is failure to admit your sleep need to yourself. It can take some time for your brain to adjust to the idea that you need less sleep than you've set as your goal. It seems very logical to conclude that being sleepy means you're not getting enough sleep. But spending too much time in bed interrupts your sleep because you exhaust your sleep drive. The daytime symptoms of spending too much time in bed are the same as the symptoms of not spending enough time in bed (tiredness, sleepiness, lack of motivation). You'll get better results if you adjust according to your sleep need.

Sometimes, it's hard to tune in to what your body is telling you. The unspoken part of CBT and CBT-I techniques is that you must pay attention to your body's cues and interpret them appropriately. If you have a history of ignoring or misinterpreting those signals, you may require assistance.

You also may be having difficulty managing anxiety and insomnia because there is another underlying problem that worsens these symptoms. There are more than 70 known sleep disorders and variations from normal sleep patterns. Most of these disorders disrupt sleep. Your difficulty with sleep may require further investigation. Some of the more common issues you may encounter are listed below.

Mind Racing

As long as you continue to pay attention to your thoughts, your mind will continue to race. When you turn your attention to something else, racing thoughts will often diminish. The tools that tend to be most helpful are mindfulness, deep breathing, muscle relaxation, and guided imagery techniques. With mindfulness, you shift your focus to what is occurring in the here and now. Deep breathing, muscle relaxation, and guided imagery help you focus and release your thoughts and bodily tensions. At the same time, you can focus on your body or on a place that is very calming and relaxing to you.

I Can't Change My Schedule

This part of the program is especially difficult. Before you change your sleep schedule, you must train your brain to think and believe that you really do need X number of hours of sleep. Actually adhering to your sleep schedule will help you adjust your thoughts. Reduce this task into smaller challenges. Begin with your wake time. Maintain a regular wake time first, regardless of how much or how little sleep you got. Always get up at the same time, seven days per week. When you become confident about waking up without hitting the snooze button, your bedtime may fall into place. Remember, it takes at least two weeks for the brain to determine that you're regulating your sleep schedule. Once you've developed a schedule, monitor how you feel and record your progress in your journal.

Sleep Restriction Isn't Working

First, you need to ask yourself if there are any other sleep hygiene issues that require adjustment. If so, begin working on those. If not, are you too tired, or are you continuing to have difficulty getting to sleep and staying asleep? In chapter 5 (see page 73), I provided suggestions about how to adjust your sleep time. Try these techniques and see if you can find your ideal sleep need.

Limiting Screen Time

We've become so dependent on our screens that it's sometimes hard to stop using them. Is there anything that you do that calms and relaxes you other than screens? Some people find reading; listening to music, podcasts, or books on tape; meditating; or praying to be calming and relaxing. Doing a puzzle can be calming. Coloring can be very relaxing. Whatever you choose, substitute screen time with one of those choices. Reward yourself for adhering to the program because this is one of the more difficult habits to change.

Waking in the Night

If this problem persists, you may need to reduce your time in bed by the amount of time you are awake in the night. Do you find it hard to go back to sleep when you wake up in the night? That could be a symptom of another sleep problem. Adjust your sleep schedule, give it at least two weeks, and see how you feel. If returning to sleep is difficult, deep breathing in bed or progressive muscle relaxation may help.

Sleep Studies

Sleep studies are most commonly performed when sleep apnea is suspected. If you snore, are a man aged 45 or older or a woman who has gone through menopause, are younger and overweight or obese, or have difficulty staying asleep or returning to sleep when you wake in the night, you may be at risk of having sleep apnea. You should consult a sleep specialist to determine your risk. If they order a sleep study, you may have an overnight study done at a sleep center, or you may be eligible for an in-home sleep apnea test. The in-center study is the first step in testing for most sleep disorders, and the in-home sleep apnea test is only indicated for sleep apnea.

Depending on the severity of sleep apnea, you'll be prescribed a treatment to facilitate breathing during sleep. If another disorder is suspected or found, further testing may be required. If insomnia persists despite use of CBT-I techniques, a sleep study also may be ordered to determine if there is another problem that impacts sleep.

GETTING SUPPORT ·····························

You now have the tools to begin resolving your anxiety and insomnia. Be patient with yourself as you implement these tools. Changing your response to anxiety and sleep habits is a challenging process. Remember to reward and congratulate yourself, even with small successes. Some of the habits you're changing have been lifelong responses to life situations, so it will take some time to change them.

CBT and CTB-I techniques are not perfect ways of dealing with anxiety and insomnia, but, for the majority of individuals, these tools can help considerably. Our sleep need typically doesn't change much over the course of our lives once we reach adulthood. However, the architecture of sleep can change, which can cause us to think we aren't sleeping well when we are really sleeping very similarly to others our age. When we are sleepy or fatigued, sometimes we don't have the mental energy to put into this process. It's okay to take a break and gather energy to tackle the issues again. Give yourself permission and time to adjust. Some can make these changes easily, while others struggle at first and, with time, their ability to use these tools improves. For a few, it's a constant struggle. If you have been using the CBT and CBT-I tools and you feel like you need help, consider enlisting the help of family, friends, or professionals.

Friends and family can help in many ways. The people who know you best may be able to help you recognize your anxiety triggers when you're not able to see them in yourself. If they know about your process, they can help by suggesting a tool to try as your mind may sometimes have difficulty grasping the tools at your disposal when you're in the midst of intrusive or negative thoughts.

Sometimes, you've put as much effort as you can into the process and need the guidance of a professional. There's no shame in getting help from a therapist. Remember, the fact that you are seeking help shows that you're committed to and invested in resolving your issues. Therapy can also be a resource for you. Therapists often have additional tools at their disposal to help with anxiety. In addition, they also have activity options that will help train your brain to avoid intrusive thoughts.

If you have been able to resolve your anxiety but your insomnia remains and you'd like assistance, find a sleep specialist with whom you can work. These individuals can guide you by pointing out some of the behavioral details that may be impairing your sleep. They'll also know when it's time for you to be further evaluated if you are making poor progress.

Regardless of where you are, continue using the techniques discussed in this book, especially if they're working. Also, remember that you'll see gradual progress with this process. The amount of time it takes to change the tracks in your brain and to change your behaviors to enhance sleep depends a great deal on how much effort you're able to put into the program. In general, it takes at least two weeks to begin feeling better. Each time you refine your sleep hygiene schedule, or change how you use sleep-interfering substances, you'll see a subtle but positive shift in your ability to get to sleep and stay asleep. Each time you use CBT techniques and notice less anxiety before bedtime, you'll see a positive change in your sleep efficiency. There is always hope for feeling better when you're doing something about the problem.

APPENDIX

. . .

The Sleep Self-Assessment

Sometimes, the patterns in our lives are not ideal for helping us get to sleep or stay asleep. This assessment will help you pinpoint the habits that may be impairing your sleep and set goals for better sleep later.

Answer the following questions to determine what your sleep and sleep habits have been like for the past month.

1. What time did you go to bed? If it varies, provide a range of times. _____

2. Is your bedroom cool, quiet, dark, and comfortable? _____

3. How long did it take you to fall asleep? If it varies, provide a range of times. _____

4. How many times did you wake up in the night? Did you get out of bed each time? _____

5. How long did it take you to return to sleep? If it varies, provide a range of times. _____

6. What time did you wake up? If it varies, provide a range of times. _____

7. On a scale of 1 to 10 (where 1 is extremely sleepy and 10 is fully rested), how did you feel on awakening in the morning on most days? _____

8. Did you take a sleeping pill or an over-the-counter sleep aid to get to sleep? _____

9. Did you drink caffeinated beverages to stay energized during the day? If so, did you drink them within eight hours of bedtime? _____

10. Did you drink alcohol within four hours of bedtime? _____

11. Do you do anything in bed other than sleep or activities relating to intimacy or sickness? _____

12. Do you turn off screens one hour before bedtime? _____

13. Do you engage in a nightly bedtime routine to prepare your body for sleep?
_____

14. Do you feel like your mind races at bedtime or when you wake in the night, making it difficult to return to sleep? _____

15. Do you watch the clock in the night? If so, do you find yourself calculating how much time you have left to sleep until your scheduled wake time? _____

16. Do you get anxious or frustrated because you cannot return to sleep? _____

17. Do you nap? If so, how long are your naps, and what time of day do you typically nap? _____

18. Does pain or stress interfere with your ability to get to sleep or stay asleep? _____

19. Do you have environmental factors that interfere with sleep (i.e., children, pets, being on call for work, noisy neighbors)? _____

20. Do you feel the need to cancel planned activities due to sleepiness or fatigue? _____

The Insomnia Severity Assessment

This assessment measures how being sleepy or tired is affecting your daily life and ability to function. Each question should be answered with a number from 1 to 4, as shown below, to describe the difficulty you have with each task as a result of sleepiness or tiredness. Place N/A in the blank if the question does not apply to you.

1 - YES, EXTREME DIFFICULTY

2 - YES, MODERATE DIFFICULTY

3 - YES, A LITTLE DIFFICULTY

4 - NO DIFFICULTY

1. Do you have difficulty concentrating on the things you do because you are sleepy or tired? _____

2. Do you have difficulty remembering things because you are sleepy or tired? _____

3. Do you have difficulty working on a hobby because you are sleepy or tired? _____

4. Do you have difficulty doing housework because you are sleepy or tired? _____

5. Do you have difficulty operating a motor vehicle for *short* distances (fewer than 100 miles) because you are sleepy or tired? _____

6. Do you have difficulty operating a motor vehicle for *long* distances (more than 100 miles) because you are sleepy or tired? _____

7. Do you have difficulty getting things done because you are too tired or sleepy to drive or take public transportation? _____

8. Do you have difficulty taking care of financial affairs and doing paperwork because you are sleepy or tired? _____

9. Do you have difficulty performing employed or volunteer work because you are too sleepy or tired? _____

10. Do you have difficulty visiting with your family or friends in *their* homes because you become sleepy or tired? _____

11. Do you have difficulty doing things for your family or friends because you are too sleepy or tired? _____

12. Has your relationship with family, friends, or work colleagues been affected because you are sleepy or tired? _____

13. Do you have difficulty exercising or participating in a sporting activity because you are too sleepy or tired? _____

14. Do you have difficulty watching a movie or video because you become sleepy or tired? _____

15. Do you have difficulty watching TV because you are sleepy or tired? _____

16. Do you have difficulty being as active as you want in the *evening* because you are too sleepy or tired? _____

17. Do you have difficulty being as active as you want in the *morning* because you are too sleepy or tired? _____

18. Do you have difficulty being as active as you want in the *afternoon* because you are too sleepy or tired? _____

19. Has your intimate or sexual relationship been affected because you are sleepy or tired? _____

20. Has your desire for intimacy or sex been affected because you are sleepy or tired? _____

To calculate your score, simply add up your answers and divide by the number of questions you answered. This will give you a number between 1 and 4. The result can be read as follows:

0 to 1.5 – Extreme dysfunction

1.6 to 2.5 – Moderate dysfunction

2.6 to 3.5 – Mild dysfunction

3.6 to 4 – No dysfunction

(Adapted from FOSQ, Weaver, 1997)

Sleep Log

		Complete this Section After Getting Out of Bed						Complete at End of Day		
Day and date	Unusual stressors: time of Alcohol & sleep medication	Time you went to bed	Time it took you to fall asleep	# of awakenings	Amount of time awake	Time you got up for the day	Total sleep time	Sleepiness Rating (see below)	Fatigue Rating	Napping: time of day & sleep amount

*Amount of time awake: this is all the time you spent awake during the night, from the first time you awakened to the time you got out of bed. It does not include the time it took you to fall asleep initially.

Sleepiness and Fatigue Rating Scale: (Average Rating for the Whole Day Following A Given Sleep Episode)

	0	25	50	75	100
SLEEPINESS:	Extremely Sleepy	Sleepy	Neither	Alert	Very Alert
FATIGUE:	Extremely Fatigued	Fatigued	Neither	Energetic	Very Energetic

RESOURCES

· · · · ·

BOOKS ·

Martin, Paul. *Counting Sheep: The Science and Pleasures of Sleep and Dreams*. New York: St. Martin's Press, 2002.

Walker, Matthew. *Why We Sleep: Unlocking the Power of Sleep and Dreams*. New York: Scribner, 2017.

APPS ·

Buddhify

Calm

CBT-I Coach

Guided Mind

Insight Timer

Sleep Diary

REFERENCES

Barrett, Lisa Feldman. *How Emotions Are Made: The Secret Life of the Brain.* New York: Houghton Mifflin Harcourt, 2017.

Beck, Judith. *Cognitive Behavior Therapy: Basics and Beyond,* 2nd Edition. New York: Guilford Press, 2011.

Benson, Herbert. *The Relaxation Response.* New York: Avon, 1957.

Calcagno, Manuel, et al. "The Thermal Effect of Food: A Review." In *Journal of the American College of Nutrition* 38, no. 6 (April 2019): 547-51.

Chellappa, Sarah, et al. "Acute Exposure to Evening Blue-Enriched Light Impacts on Human Sleep." In *Journal of Sleep Research* 22, no. 5 (October 2013): 573-80.

Clark, David, and Aaron Beck. *The Anxiety & Worry Workbook: The Cognitive Behavioral Solution.* New York: Guilford Press, 2012.

Dement, William. *The Promise of Sleep.* New York: Dell Publishing, 1999.

Edinger, J. D., et al. "A Cognitive-Behavioral Therapy for Sleep-Maintenance Insomnia in Older Adults." In *Psychology and Aging* 7, no. 2 (June 1992): 282-9.

Epstein, Lawrence. *The Harvard Medical School Guide to A Good Night's Sleep.* New York: McGraw Hill, 2007.

Forman, Evan, et al. "A Randomized Controlled Effectiveness Trial of Acceptance and Commitment Therapy and Cognitive Therapy for Anxiety and Depression." In *Behavior Modification*. November 1, 2007. https://doi.org/10.1177/0145445507302202.

Fournier, Debra. "Anxiety Disorders." In *Primary Care: A Collaborative Practice*, eds. Terry Buttaro, et al. St. Louis: Mosby, 2013.

Gillihan, Seth. *Cognitive Behavioral Therapy Made Simple: 10 Strategies for Managing Anxiety, Depression, Anger, Panic, and Worry*. Emeryville: Althea Press, 2018.

Goodheart, Annette. *Laughter Therapy: How to Laugh About Everything in Your Life That Isn't Really Funny*. Santa Barbara: Less Stress Press, 1994

Hall, John. *Guyton and Hall Textbook of Medical Physiology*. Philadelphia: Saunders, 2011.

Hirschkowitz, Max, et al. "The National Sleep Foundation's Sleep Time and Duration Recommendations: Methodology and Results Summary." In *Sleep Health* 1, no. 1 (March 2015): 40-43.

Jayakody, Kaushadh, et al. "Exercise for Anxiety Disorders: A Systematic Review." In *British Journal of Sports Medicine* 48, no. 3 (February 2014): 187-96.

King, Brian. *The Habits of Stress-Resilient People*. Seminar presented in Nashville, TN on October 15, 2019.

King, Brian. *The Laughing Cure: Emotional and Physical Healing—A Comedian Reveals Why Laughter Really Is the Best Medicine*. New York: Skyhorse Publishing, 2016.

Ko, Hae-Jin, and Chang-Ho Youn. "Effects of Laughter Therapy on Depression, Cognition, and Sleep Among the Community-Dwelling Elderly." In

Geriatrics & Gerontology International 11, no. 3. Accessed November 23, 2019. https://doi.org/10.1111/j.1447-0594.2010.00680.x.

Mackay, Graham, and James Neill. "The Effect of 'Green' Exercise on State Anxiety and the Role of Exercise Duration, Intensity and Greenness: A Quasi-Experimental Study." In *Psychology of Sport and Exercise* 11, no. 3. (May 2010): 238-45.

Martin, Paul. *Counting Sheep: The Science and Pleasures of Sleep and Dreams.* New York: St. Martin's Press, 2002.

Mayo Clinic. "Psychotherapy." https://www.mayoclinic.org/tests -procedures/psychotherapy/about/pac-20384616 on 11/10/2019.

McLeod, Saul. "Cognitive Behavioral Therapy." In *Simply Psychology.* Updated 2019. https://www.simplypsychology.org/cognitive-therapy.html.

Milewski, Matthew, et al. "Chronic Lack of Sleep is Associated with Increased Sports Injuries in Adolescent Athletes." In *Journal of Paediatric Orthopaedics* 34, no. 2 (March 2014): 129-33.

Robson, David. "How We Could Sleep Better in Less Time" In *BBC: Work Life.* November 25, 2019. https://www.bbc.com/worklife/article/20191122 -how-to-sleep-better.

Roth, Thomas. "Insomnia: Definition, Prevalence, Etiology, and Conse- quences." In *Journal of Clinical Sleep Medicine* 3 Supplement, no. 5 (August 2007) S7-S10.

Sateia, Michael, ed. *International Classification of Sleep Disorders*, 3rd Edition. Darien: American Academy of Sleep Medicine, 2014.

Sinngareddy, Ravi, et al. "Fatigue or Daytime Sleepiness?" In *Journal of Clini- cal Sleep Medicine* 6, no. 4 (August 15, 2010): 405.

Titov, N., et al. "Disorder-Specific Versus Transdiagnostic and Clinician-Guided Versus Self-Guided Treatment for Major Depressive Disorder and Comorbid Anxiety Disorders: A Randomized Controlled Trial." In *Journal of Anxiety Disorders* 35 (October 2015) 88-102.

Tochikubo, Osamu, et al. "Effects of Insufficient Sleep on Blood Pressure Monitored by a New Multibiomedical Recorder." In *Hypertension* 27, no. 6 (1996): 1318-24.

Walker, Matthew. *Why We Sleep: Unlocking the Power of Sleep and Dreams.* New York: Scribner, 2017.

Weaver, Terri. "Functional Outcomes of Sleep Questionnaire." 1996.

Wignall, Nick. "Cognitive Restructuring: The Complete Guide to Changing Negative Thinking." In *Better Thinking, Emotional Fitness.* April 8, 2019. https://nickwignall.com/cognitive-restructuring/.

INDEX

· · · · ·

ACKNOWLEDGEMENTS

· · · · · · · · · · · · · · · · · · · ·

I would like to thank my manager, Amber O'Neil, my son, Brandon Bowers, and my mentor, Kelly Carden, for their help with ideas on how to present parts of this work and their support as I engaged in the writing process. In addition, I would like to thank my sister, Carol Deterding, for her emotional support as I was writing this book.

ABOUT THE AUTHOR

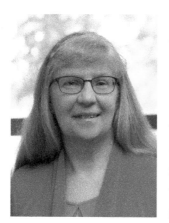

Renata Alexandre is a certified nurse practitioner who holds a PhD in health and human performance and has master's degrees in nursing, divinity, and sociology. Clinically, her passion is sleep medicine. She is an expert in diagnosing and treating all of the seventy-four known sleep disorders. She has specialized training in cognitive behavioral therapy for insomnia (CBT-I). Alexandre also has expertise in tailoring treatment for patients' individual needs, including medication selection and weaning or reducing doses of sleep aids. She has more than a decade of clinical experience in sleep medicine.

CPSIA information can be obtained
at www.ICGtesting.com
Printed in the USA
LVHW051613280320
651414LV00002B/2